A HISTORY OF MEDICINE

BRIAN INGLIS

A HISTORY OF

MEDICINE

THE WORLD PUBLISHING COMPANY 31,89

CLEVELAND AND NEW YORK

Published by The World Publishing Company
2231 West 110th Street, Cleveland 2, Ohio

R 131
I 55
(1.)

Library of Congress Catalog Card Number: 65–24165

Copyright © 1965 by Brian Inglis
Printed in Great Britain by Morrison & Gibb Ltd London and Edinburgh
Illustrations printed by Jarrolds of Norwich

CONTENTS

CONTENTS

ILLUSTRATIONS

Taking the pulse, from Cleyer's *Specimen medicinae Sinicae*
Ivory model used by Chinese ladies for describing their illnesses. Department of the
History of Medicine, University of Kansas Medical Center

EGYPT (*between pages 24 and 25*)

Relief of Hesy-ré on a wooden panel from his tomb at Saqqâra. Third dynasty (2778–
2723 BC) (*Photo: Hirmer Fotoarchiv*)
Part of a page from the Ebers Papyrus, from a facsimile in *Papyros Ebers, das hermetische
Buch über die Arzeneimittel der alten Ägypter in hieratischer Schrift*, edited by Georg
Ebers. Leipzig, 1875
Aknahton with his wife and children; limestone relief from his palace at Tell el Amarna
(*c.* 1360 BC). Ägyptische Abteilung der Staatlichen Museen, Berlin
Nefertiti offering Aknahton a mandrake plant. Ägyptische Abteilung der Staatlichen
Museen, Berlin

GREECE (*between pages 24 and 25*)

Maenads dancing in an orgiastic rite at a wine-festival; from an Attic stamnos by the
Dinos painter (*c.* 420 BC). Museo Nazionale, Naples (*Photo: Hirmer Fotoarchiv*)
Chiron, Thetis and Peleus, from an Attic black-figure vase (*c.* 510 BC). Museum Antiker
Kleinkunst, Munich
Relief of Archinos dedicated to Amphiaros, divine oracle of Oropos (*c.* 380–370 BC).
National Museum, Athens (*Photo: German Archeological Institute, Athens*)
Aesculapius and Hygeia, from an ivory diptych (*c.* AD 400). City of Liverpool Museums
Hippocrates from a Byzantine manuscript of his works (*c.* 1342). Bibliothèque Nationale,
ms. gr. 2144, fol. 10v. (*Photo: Hirmer Fotoarchiv*)
Miniature from a tenth-century manuscript of Nicandor's *Theriaca*. Bibliothèque
Nationale, ms. suppl. gr. 247, fol. 47v. (*Photo: Hirmer Fotoarchiv*)
Miniature from a fourteenth-century manuscript of the *Antidotarium* of Myrepsos.
Bibliothèque Nationale, ms. gr. 2243, fol. 10v.

ROME (*between pages 40 and 41*)

Japyx treats Aeneas with Dittamy collected by Venus on Mount Ida; fresco from
Pompeii. Museo Nazionale, Naples (*Photo: Alinari*)
Ruins of the Baths of Caracalla (*Photo: Min. Aeronautica U.S.P. – Alinari*)
Reconstruction of wall-decoration in the Baths of Titus, from *Description des Bains de
Titus, ou collection de peintures trouvées dans les ruines des thermes de cet Empereur . . .* by
Nicolas Ponce. Paris, 1786
Pont du Gard (*Photo: French Government Tourist Office*)
Gallo-Roman relief depicting an apothecary. Musée d'Épinal (*Photo: Archives Photo-
graphiques*)

ILLUSTRATIONS

PLAGUES AND EPIDEMICS (*between pages 72 and 73*)

Three doctors attending a plague patient from *Das buch zu distillieren die zusamen gethonen ding Composita genant, durch die eintzigē ding* . . . by Hieronymus Brunschwig. Strasbourg, 1519

St Roch from a plague sheet (Rhineland, *c.* 1470) from Heitz's *Pestblätter*. Original in the Biblioteca Classense, Ravenna

Burial of plague victims at Tournai in 1349 from the Annals of Gilles le Muisit. Bibliothèque Royale, Brussels, ms. 13076/7, fol. 24v

Woodcut illustration by Hans Weiditz to the *Trotspiegel in Glück und Unglück Francisci Petrarchae* . . . Frankfurt, 1620

Title-page to the *Regimen zu deutsch Magistri philippi Culmachers vō Eger wider die grausamen erschrecklichen Totlichen pestilentz* . . . Leipzig, 1495 (?)

Plague sheet invoking St Sebastian, fron Linange, Lorraine (early sixteenth-century); from Heitz's *Pestblätter*. Original in the Stadtbibliothek, Schlettstadt

Doctor visiting a plague patient; illustration by Gentile Bellini to the *Fascicolo de medicina in Volgare* . . . (by John de Ketham). Venice, 1493

The Baths of Leuk, Valais (1597) by Hans Bock the elder. Oeffentliche Kunstsammlung, Basle

Illustrations of two witches from *De Lanijs et phitoicis* [sic. i.e. lamiis et pythonicis] *mulieribus* . . . *tractatus pulcherrimus* by Ulrich Molitor de Constantia. Cologne, 1490 (?)

Two Witches (1523) by Hans Baldung Grien. Städelsches Kunstinstitut, Frankfurt

Pilgrimage of Epileptics to Meulebeke (1564) by Pieter Brueghel the elder. Albertina, Vienna (*Photo: Bildarchiv der österreichischen Nationalbibliothek*)

Alsatian plague sheet (*c.* 1480) invoking St Valentine of Rufach, from Heitz's *Pestblätter*. Original formerly in the Paul Heitz collection, Strasbourg

THE RENAISSANCE (*between pages 88 and 89*)

Anatomy Lesson of Mundinus at Padua; illustration by Gentile Bellini to Ketham's *Fascicolo*

Anatomy Lesson from a fifteenth-century Latin manuscript of Avicenna's *De Medicina*. Hunterian Library, Glasgow, ms. 9, fol. 22

Illustration of a dissection from *Le proprietaire des choses* by Bartholomaeus Anglicus. Lyons, 1482

Anatomia ossium corporis humani by Richard Hela (Nuremberg, 1493) from *Holzschnitte aus dem ersten und zweiten Drittel des fünfzehnten Jahrhunderts in der Kgl. Graphischen Sammlung zu München* by W. L. Schreiber. Strasbourg, 1912

Tree of the Vessels by Leonardo da Vinci (Quaderni d' Anatomia V, fol. 1). Royal Library, Windsor Castle (reproduced by Gracious Permission of Her Majesty the Queen)

John Banister's Anatomy Lesson (1581). Hunterian Library, Glasgow

Portrait of Ambroise Paré from *Les Œuures d'Ambroise Paré* . . . *Reueuz & augmentez par l'autheur, pour la seconde edition*. Paris, 1579

THE EIGHTEENTH CENTURY (*between pages 120 and 121*)

SURGERY AND HOSPITALS (*between pages 136 and 137*)

Illustration from *Facts in Mesmerism* . . . C. H. Townshend. London, 1840

Illustration by George Du Maurier for his book *Trilby*. London, 1895

Advertisement for sessions of magnetism and somnambulism (Paris, mid-nineteenth century). Musée Carnavalet, Paris (*Photo: René-Jacques*)

Photographs of a woman in a hypnotic trance from *Nouvelle iconographie de la Salpêtrière. Clinique des maladies du système nerveux. Publiées sous la direction du Professeur Charcot . . . tome IV*. Paris, 1891

Charcot lecturing at the Salpêtrière. E. P. Goldschmidt and Co, London

Photograph of man suffering from persecution mania, from *Nouvelle iconographie de la Salpêtrière . . . tome VIII*, 1895

PUBLIC HEALTH AND MODERN DRUGS (*between pages 168 and 169*)

Hand of Sarah Nelmes infected with cowpox, from *An Inquiry into the causes and effects of the variolae vaccinae, a disease discovered in some of the Western Counties of England . . . known by the name of the cow pox* by Edward Jenner. London, 1798

The Cow Pock – or – the Wonderful Effects of The New Inoculation! by James Gillray. London, 1802. Wellcome Historical Medical Museum

The Naples Health Office from *Lazarettos in Europe: with various pages relative to the Plague: together with further observations on some foreign prisons and hospitals . . .* by John Howard. Warrington, 1789

Barrack kitchen at Scutari, from *Soyer's Culinary Campaign . . . With the plain art of cookery for military and civil institutions, the army, navy, public etc.* London, 1857

Thermal baths at Caldas de Reinha. Camera Municipal, Lisbon (*Photo: Mario Novais*)

Miss Kennedy distributing clothing at Kilrush during the Irish Famine of 1849. From the *Illustrated London News*. (*Photo: Mansell Collection*)

Plague-spot at South Lambeth in 1843 (*Photo: Radio Times Hulton Picture Library*)

Photograph of Newcastle slums, *c.* 1880 (*Photo: Radio Times Hulton Picture Library*)

Road-Sweeper at Chandigarh, India (*Photo: T. S. Satyan – World Health Organisation*)

Nigerian women crowding to be given a drug for protection against meningitis (*Photo: D. Henrioud – World Health Organisation*)

Nigerian child with yaws before and after a penicillin injection (*Photo: Eric Schwab – World Health Organisation*)

Children in Taiwan queuing up for inoculation (*Photo: World Health Organisation*)

Collection of modern drugs (*Photo: © Topix copyright by Thomson Newspapers*)

Cartoon by J. W. Taylor from the author's collection (reproduced by permission of *Punch*)

ENDPAPERS

The Physician's Visit by Abraham Bosse. British Museum

ILLUSTRATIONS

COLOUR ILLUSTRATIONS

The author and publishers would like to thank the institutions and photographers mentioned above for kind permission to use their photographs. Photographs from the Wellcome Historical Medical Museum and Library are reproduced by courtesy of the Wellcome Trustees.

Photographs from books, unless otherwise credited, were taken by J. R. Freeman and Co from copies in the British Museum or the Library of the Royal College of Surgeons of England (by courtesy of the President and Council).

The layout of the illustrations is by Arthur T. Lockwood.

INTRODUCTION

MOST of us grow up to regard health as the natural, and disease as an unnatural, state of man; so much so that theologians have had to devote much anxious thought to explaining why the gods should have adopted what seems such an arbitrary, unfair and cruel form of retribution – for how else can it be accounted for? But looked at as an evolutionary expedient, disease becomes understandable: nature has invented and exploited it to ease her selection problems, to enable the fittest to survive.

Three main types of disease with an evolutionary purpose can be observed in animal life. There is constitutional defect, or deficiency – a way of reducing or eliminating weaker strains. There are the degenerative disorders, related to the process of ageing and eventually dying – almost as if animals which become expendable are being nudged into earlier completion of their life cycle to make room for others. And there are diseases caused by failure to master enemies. We make a distinction between being killed by a lion or by a microbe – the one being regarded as death by misadventure, the other as succumbing to a disease; but both can be attributed to nature's design to preserve the balance of the species.

There is, however, a distinction: whereas the lion kills deliberately, for food, microbes may have no direct interest in the death of the animal or human in whom they find themselves. Quite the reverse, for basically they are parasites; and to the parasite – microbe or flea, tapeworm or sucking-fish – the host's death is usually inconvenient and can be fatal. As Zinsser pointed out in his *Rats, Lice and History*, nature has been extremely logical: for the price of some loss of liberty she has offered parasites a release from the necessity to work, from uncertainty and from exposure, a secure and effortless existence on an island of plenty; 'by adapting itself to parasitism the louse has attained the ideal of bourgeois civilisation, though its methods are more direct than those of business or banking, and its source of nourishment is not its own species'. But the bourgeoisie (Zinsser was writing in the 1930s, when both the term and its derogatory connotation were more fashionable) did not deliberately invest their wealth in dying concerns, which is what microbes are continually doing.

Why, then, should they cause disease? The answer is that they do not: they happen to be the agents of disease, through no choice of their own. The ideal of any parasite is to come to terms with its host, so that the two can live amicably – or at least without the kind of friction that will weaken the host, reducing his chances of survival. But in certain circumstances microbes become dangerous to their hosts, and to themselves. Some of them may be likened to members of a fifth column, who lead outwardly respectable lives until they receive orders to foment a rising; others, to those normally law-abiding citizens who, when law and order break down, emerge as looters.

But again, why? We do not know: but the probability is that nature has allowed them to adopt parasitism as a way of life on these terms. It is as if the directive had run 'you can enjoy the good life, but only so long as it suits nature's evolutionary purpose. At some point, she may issue instructions that your host species must be culled; and then, you will be called upon to do it.' That, at least, seems the most likely explanation of infectious diseases, and their spread by epidemics, when parasites which have been leading a harmless existence suddenly break out and go on the rampage.

The process can be observed in human beings (most of us are 'carriers' of flu viruses, but we do not continually suffer from flu); and it is sometimes possible in a laboratory to change the character of a micro-organism from Hyde to Jekyll, and back again. How the signal is given in nature remains a mystery; but so far as can be judged by fossil remains, this evolutionary expedient was adopted at a very early stage.

Animals have always suffered from diseases, and very much the same kind of disease which they – and we – suffer from today. This even includes the kind of disorders which, when they afflict humans, we describe as mental; the best known example being the one which affects lemmings. Lemmings inexplicably commit what used to be regarded as mass suicide, every few years; they rush down the Scandinavian hillsides, like the Gadarene swine, until they reach lakes, or fjords, and then swim out to drown. The suicide, though, is not deliberate. What they are really engaged in – it is now believed – is

2

migration; when a stretch of water faces them, they try to swim across it, and they drown because they are caught in a storm, or have insufficient endurance. Migration is commonly a protective device in nature; some animals instinctively change their habitat for sensible reasons, to take advantage of a better climate or diet. But in the lemmings' case, it appears to be a rough-and-ready method of regulating their numbers. When lemming stocks increase to the point when overpopulation becomes a danger to the community as a whole, some of them are afflicted by a kind of mass hysteria, producing a character change. From being timid and cautious, they grow bold, and even aggressive; setting out like vikings to conquer new territory, showing fight where ordinarily they would hide. But nature has deceived them: their migration leads them not to a lemming El Dorado, but to death.

This is the hypothesis – admittedly still speculative, because it is impossible to be certain that the lemmings' change of character is the cause of the move; it might conceivably be the consequence. Still, the most likely explanation is that it represents an automatic safety valve; when a certain degree of over-crowding is imminent, the psychological release mechanism operates, to protect the community at the expense of some of its members. Of course the process may be found to be 'physical', in the sense that the release may be prompted by some biochemical change – as it may also be in schizophrenia. But this would not disturb the hypothesis that the disorder has an evolutionary purpose.

Disease, then, however unpleasant for the recipient, is designed for the ultimate benefit of the species. The trouble is that the evolutionary method is inefficient – unrefined. Sometimes it works satisfactorily for years; when rabbits are in an environment where they have few natural enemies – on an island, say – disease may regularly kill off just enough of them to keep the population stable, and prevent their numbers from expanding until they starve. But should a new virus be introduced, they may be wiped out altogether. Epidemics then, although they are part of the evolutionary mechanism, are also an example of its imperfections.

To preserve nature's balance, evolution had also to provide some counter to disease; and the main instrument which it perfected was the built-in recuperative power which the Hippocratic writings called *vis medicatrix naturae*: the life force. 'Life force' is not an ideal translation, as colloquially it can embrace

3

anything from the act of breathing to an abstraction like 'the will to live'; but in a medical context it is usually applied to those measures which are taken automatically in animal life, even down to the earthworm level, to repair damage, or to throw off the effects of poisons. A cut will heal, if left alone; a broken bone will knit together again; through sneezing, or vomiting, or sealing up in a boil, unwelcome microbes or toxic substances can be expelled.

To prevent the balance being upset by destructive epidemics, animal bodies became capable of learning by experience. When a small-scale attack by a specific virus was beaten off, the body's defences were able to profit from the encounter, and could defeat much heavier attacks in future. So successful was this immunisation process that the scales might even have become too heavily weighted against the disease agents, but they had one considerable advantage – biological flexibility. Because generation succeeds generation every half hour or so, the microbes' rate of evolutionary development is formidable. So although diseases have changed relatively little down the millennia, they have never remained static: new disease agents are constantly emerging, or old ones changing their character, presenting the hosts with fresh problems.

The life force also evolved ingenious ways of resisting the threat of disease agents: instinct, for one. Zoologists frequently turn up examples of the way in which animals who are in danger of suffering from a dietary deficiency will travel long distances to find what their bodies lack. Professor Ritchie Calder has collected more curious instances: 'sheep with a diet deficient in lime have been known to eat, with geometrical exactitude, the grass of a squared plot which had been limed, before turning to other pastures which would satisfy their hunger but lacked the subtler medical requirements. On a South African veldt, cattle were dying of a mysterious epidemic. One group survived and it was found that they were eating the bark and herbage of a tree in the trunk of which there was a single copper nail. The rest of the cattle were sick from a deficiency of minute traces of copper.' The earthworm can reconstitute itself into two earthworms after it has been cut in half by a spade; the lizard can grow a new tail; the salamander, a new limb. In what we are accustomed to regard complacently as the ascent on the evolutionary scale, certain reparative processes which would be invaluable to us have been lost. To think of man's health organisation as being on a higher level than the animals', then, is a little presumptuous.

PRIMITIVE MAN

PRIMITIVE man, as a product of the evolutionary process, was subject to the same hazards as other animals, and protected by the same reflexes and instincts. He, too, had his genetic weaknesses, his degenerative disorders and his enemies, ranging from dinosaurs to viruses: he, too, obeyed the promptings of his life force, which showed him how to maintain a reasonably balanced diet and which threw out poisons, if it could, when he absorbed them by mistake. But in some ways he was confronted with greater problems than animals. He began to walk upright, a position for which his body was not entirely suited – it made him accident- and strain-prone; and he sometimes had to seek the protection of caves, not the healthiest of dwelling places. He also underwent a change which was to exercise a profound influence on his health, as well as on the general development of the species *homo sapiens*. His cortex, the seat of his emerging reason, began to develop with (by evolutionary standards) unexampled rapidity.

Dr A. T. W. Simeons traced the influence of the developing cortex in *Man's Presumptuous Brain*. Its initial function, he suggested, was primarily as a censor, to select from the alternatives presented to it by instinct and by memory. An animal, confronted by danger, had the choice of running away; remaining still, and hoping not to be noticed; or offering fight. But the 'choice' was often dictated by whichever instinct happened to be paramount, rather than the needs of a particular situation: 'playing possum' tricked some opossum's natural enemies; now it only simplifies the task of a hunter. Primitive man, however, learned how to apply reason to make his choice, when in a predicament. He consciously estimated whether he could reach and climb a tree before being intercepted, and if not, how best he could deceive or destroy his pursuers. All this time, his instincts might be clamouring at him to fight, or to run away; but his cortex could censor them and give its own instructions to his limbs.

In evolutionary terms, this development of the reasoning faculty was a spectacular advance; but from the point of view of man's health, Simeons pointed out, it has had its disadvantages. Man 'no longer follows the dictates of biological necessity. Determining what the cortex allows into consciousness are conventions, habits and the postulates of civilisation.' And long before the postulates of civilisation began to enforce themselves, primitive man's new attribute of reason must have been prompting him to false decisions. Instinct might have warned him against eating a certain type of berry, or fungus; reason – based on memory – would recall that it had tasted very good the last time; and memory might deceive – it might have been a similar but non-poisonous species that he had enjoyed before. It was useful to primitive man to be able to remember, and record, what remedies had brought him relief in the past – what herb, say, had cured his stomach ache. But again, reason was not always a more reliable guide than instinct: pains in the stomach may come from different causes, requiring different treatment.

Inevitably, primitive man began to try to combat illness; and anthropologists have been able to study the process in tribes living in ways which are unlikely to be very different from those which characterised man in prehistoric times (attempts have been made to differentiate between 'prehistoric' and 'primitive' medicine – reasonably enough, as the attitudes and achievements of the cave man must have been very different from those of tribal communities that were to develop; but it will require a great deal more research before the distinction can be of more than academic interest).

In a few communities, primitive man practised nothing that can reasonably be described as medicine at all. There was what amounted to first aid, for cuts and bruises; minor illnesses were taken for granted, and borne until they disappeared; but serious diseases, like smallpox, were looked on simply as a menace to the community – the victim was deserted, and left to die; or to recover on his own, if he was lucky. But this seems to have been unusual. The causes of illness must have aroused speculations from very early times, as soon as man was capable of worrying about them; and out of it arose what Henry Sigerist, the greatest of medical historians, called the basic concept of disease – that it 'is a "Plus" or a "Minus"; a "Too-much" or a "Not-enough": Man is sick because there is something in his body that does not belong to it, or he is sick because something has been removed from his organism that is necessary to life.' Understandably, diseases were often attributed to the malice of enemies introducing something into, or withdrawing something from, the patient. And when those enemies were clearly not doing it openly, with a spear or with poison, they must be exploiting some means that could not be detected by the ordinary senses. They must be using magic.

The medicine man did not – and to this day does not – usually practise medicine in the ordinary sense. He practised magic, with healing his objective – though, as the assumption was that disease was caused by magic, or witchcraft, the remedy was often actually designed to harm – to kill off, or frighten off, the purveyors – man or evil spirits – in the hope that this would allow their victim to recover. Medicine men used a great variety of techniques. Perhaps the best known was imitative magic: an effigy was made of the (presumed) guilty party, and pins were stuck into it; or it was burned, or mutilated. Charms, spells, incantations, or rituals might be used to ward off sickness. Some medicine men actually used medicine – a herbal infusion, say: but even then they often sought to endow it with magic properties.

With medicine becoming increasingly rationalist, it is not surprising that most historians of medicine have been concerned to emphasise how far modern science has brought us from such primitive hocus-pocus. But a few of the more perceptive writers have cautioned against this attitude; notably Fielding H. Garrison, whose formidable *Introduction to the History of Medicine* appeared just before the First World War.

To many of Garrison's contemporaries, caught up in the growing scientific rationalism of the time, primitive medicine stood condemned because of the resemblance between the methods that the medicine man used and those of the quacks who had flourished in the late nineteenth century. But for Garrison, this resemblance was a good reason for taking medicine men seriously. They exploited superstition, certainly, but this 'can be approached in no derisive spirit, especially in the light of modern quackery and its successes. The closer we look into the ways of primitive man, the more liable it is to take down our own conceit.' Later Sigerist was to agree: 'it is an insult to the medicine man to call him the ancestor of the modern physician. He is that, to be sure, but is much more: namely the ancestor of most of our professions . . . he knows more than other people about the transcendental world, so much so that he even has power over it.'

At the time Sigerist was embarking on his history, in the 1940s, this was an unusual and bold attitude to adopt. For a scientist even to mention a 'transcendental world', let alone to appear to accept its existence, was an open invitation to ridicule. Yet since his death, research has been vindicating his judgment; in particular by demonstrating the astonishing therapeutic potential of suggestion. Primitive man must often have suffered from what would now be diagnosed as stress symptoms; and against them, suggestion has been shown to be widely effective in a way that until recently was hardly suspected. It can also exert a powerful, even if usually temporary, effect on the course of degenerative disorders. The scope, therefore, for a medicine man, even if he had no other therapeutic skill than that which his hold over other men's imaginations gave him, must have been very great.

But medicine men usually also enjoyed a secondary aid: the manipulation of the trance state. As Professor G. M. Carstairs has commented, trance states – in which the normal self appears to surrender possession of the body to an alien personality – are exceptional and rather suspect in most civilised communities; but in many parts of the world they are still common, 'being witnessed, if not actually experienced, by every member of society. These states are always regarded as having a special quality, as bringing one into closer touch with the world of spirits; and yet when they are very widespread they serve in a way to domesticate the supernatural.'

The phrase 'domesticate the supernatural' is felicitous; it precisely describes the therapeutic function of the trance. The accepted explanation has usually been that the body is harbouring an evil spirit, which can be thrown out in the course of the trance – hence the frequent accompanying convulsions. But it is not necessary to believe in evil spirits, to accept that going into and coming out of a trance state can fulfil a healing role – as abreaction or shock therapy do today. And although the old-style convulsive trance may no longer be fashionable in civilised communities, proof of the healing powers latent in it has been given by research into its more refined version – the hypnotic trance, which has been used to give many remarkable, if not always permanent, cures.

But did medicine men also, as Sigerist implied, wield healing powers which cannot be accounted for by suggestion alone, with or without the assistance of trances? A regular accompaniment of this type of healing – whether conducted by African medicine men, or by the Kahunas ('Guardians of the Mystery') in Hawaii, or by saints in Christian lore – is the assumption

8

Primitive Medicine

Paleolithic cave-painting from the Pech-Merle cave. The silhouettes of hands above the dappled horses may have been to ward off the evil eye and give protection from disease and danger

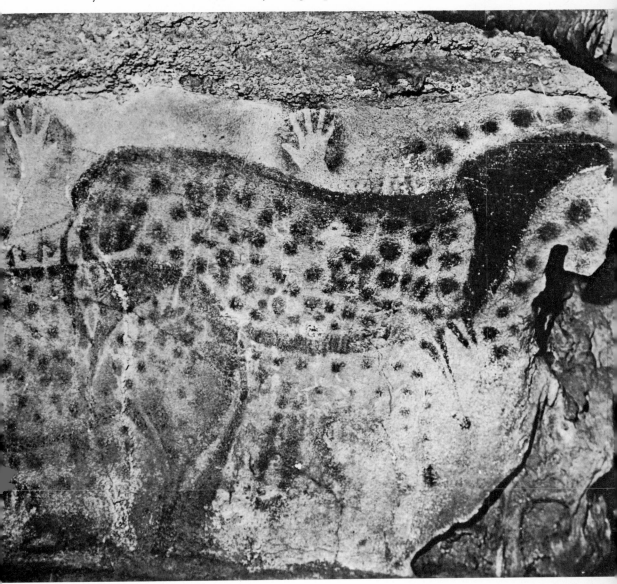

Mochica doctor from Peru
(before 1000 AD) casting a spell over
a patient, to take away his illness

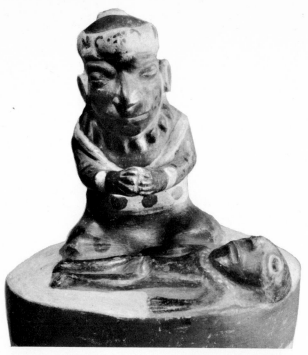

Savages from the north-east coast
of South America who cure their
sick by first forcibly dipping them
in water, then beating them round
a huge bonfire, then bleeding, and
finally putting them to rest in their
hammocks

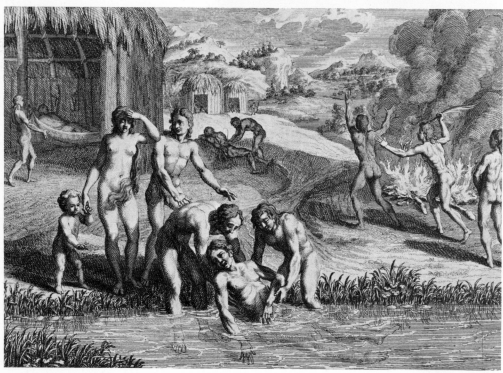

Eskimo shamans, one with the
drum used to induce the trance state
and the other in a trance drawing
the sickness out of the patient's head
with his stave

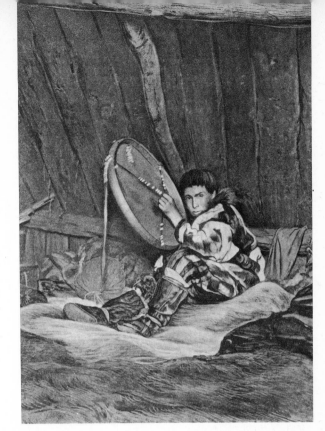

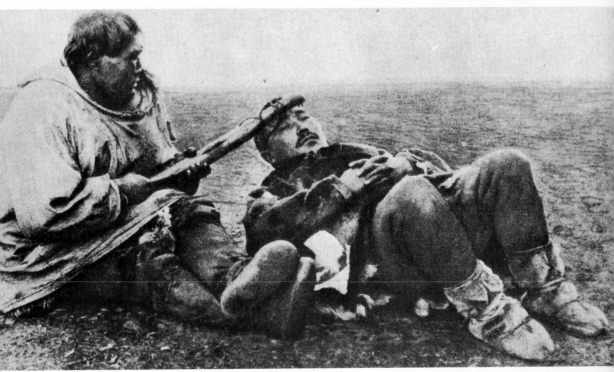

Ravâna the disease-bringing demon of the Khmers from Angkor Wat. Many primitive peoples think of disease as caused by evil spirits, and their medical practice consists of protecting themselves against them

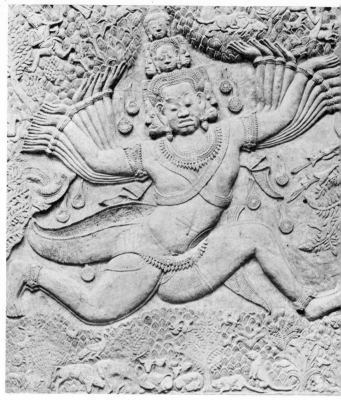

Right: African nail fetish, used as a protection against the spirits of disease

Far right: Use of the mandrake plant recurs throughout medical history. Here a forged mandrake root made in the sixteenth century has been clothed in cap and undergarment made from the skin of an unborn baby and a black silk gown, for medical or magical uses

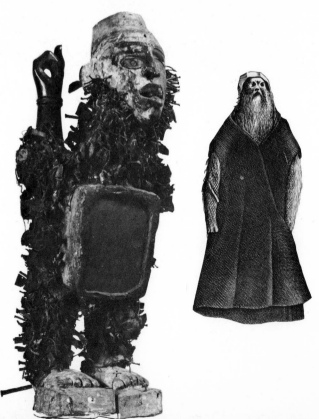

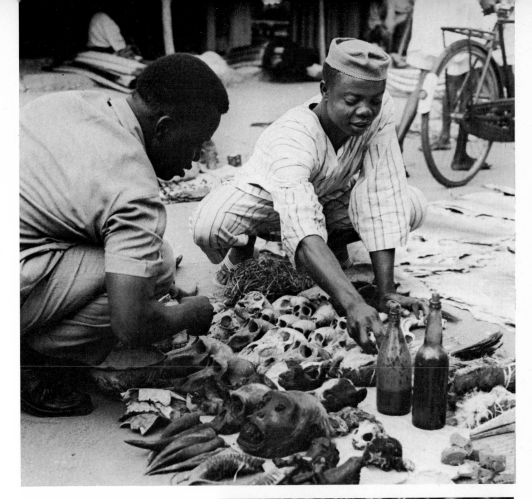

Qualified African doctor at the stall
of a man who sells dried skulls and
potions as magic protection against
disease

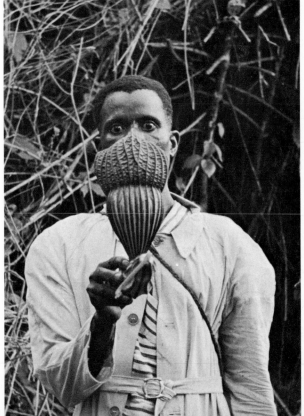

Medicine-man of the Toma tribe
from Guinea with a plant of good
omen, to be used for divination

China

Early Chinese anatomical chart, possibly of Korean origin, showing the main organs of the body. From a seventeenth-century European work on Chinese medicine

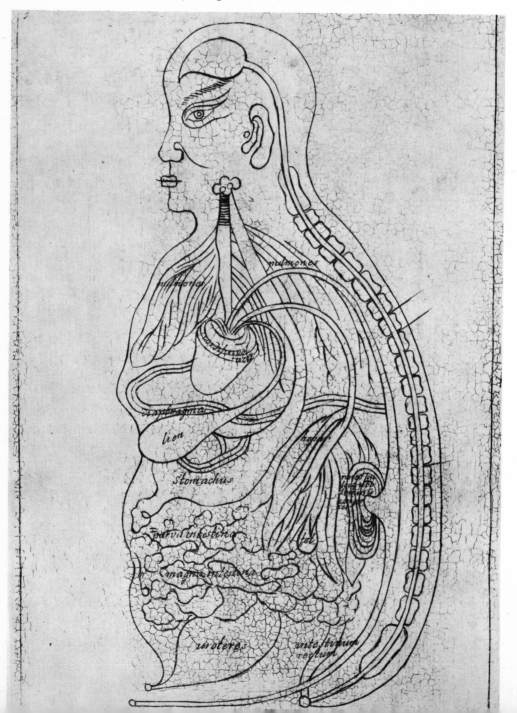

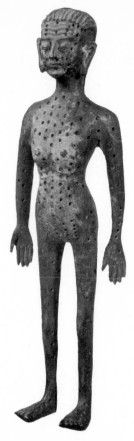

Model of a man indicating the points where the skin should be pricked by the acupuncturist's needles

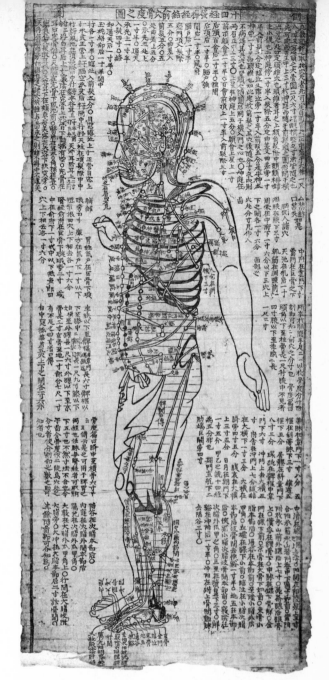

Right: One of a set of three Japanese eighteenth-century charts showing acupuncture points on the front, the back and, here, the side of the body

Japanese woman after acupuncture treatment for 'colic' depicted by Kaempffer, who travelled to Japan in the late seventeenth century

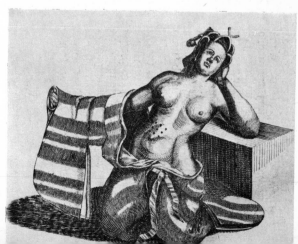

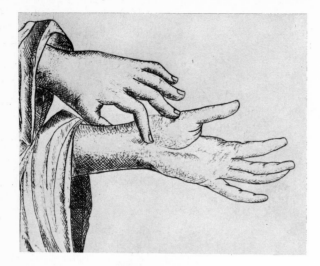

One of the methods of taking the pulse, an art brought to perfection by the Chinese, and used in conjunction with acupuncture

Ivory model used by Chinese ladies of high birth to point out in what part of their body they felt pain, since it was improper to undress in front of their doctor

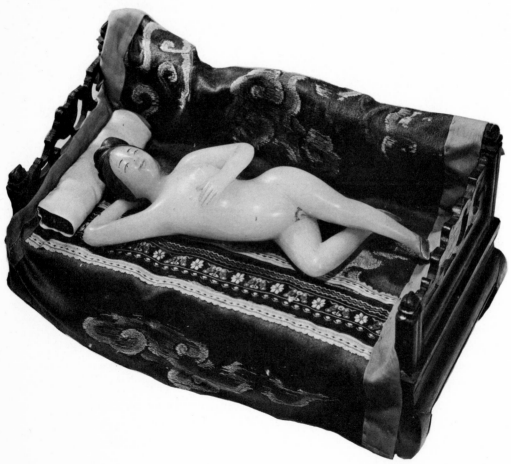

that certain individuals have power to heal at a distance, by magic or by prayer – or to harm at a distance, by sticking pins into a wax model of the enemy, or by some similar formula. Understandably, such reports tended to be scoffed at by medical scientists, because to accept them would have involved lending credence to the supernatural. Recently, however, a possible rational explanation has been put forward, relating absent healing to the transmission of suggestion by extra-sensory communication.

Although this is as yet no more than an interesting hypothesis, it ties in with the fact that much primitive healing relied for diagnosis largely on divination. Doctors were 'seers'. So far as patients were concerned, the trance state might be simply for purposes of treatment; but for the medicine man, the prime object of going into a trance was to throw off consciousness in order to 'divine' where the cause of the illness lay, much as a dowser seeks to divine where water lies. And although resistance to accepting the possibility that medicine men have actually possessed powers of divination (or even to accepting that dowsers can find water) remains quite widespread, the scientific evidence for extra-sensory transmission and perception is now strong enough to lend it respectability. Its use in healing, then – still widespread all over the world, and encountered in every era of history – may yet be explained, and shown to have been genuine (though not in all its manifestations); rather than simply a massive monument to the gullibility of man.

If the divination theory is correct, too, it helps to account for the reverence felt in many primitive communities for psychotics. Where the conscious mind is not securely established in control, the unconscious may break through from time to time; and in civilised communities, where trust is placed in rationality, this is regarded as a sign of mental affliction. But primitive communities were more inclined to place their trust in the irrational: often rightly, as reason was a less mature and consequently an even more untrustworthy guide than it is today. Psychosis, therefore, was regarded with awe, and even veneration; and the psychotic might find himself being groomed for the role of medicine man. He might be schizophrenic, or he might suffer from occasional dissociation, as mediums do: either way, the outpourings of his second self were ordinarily regarded as coming from a spirit, or a god, of a higher order than the evil spirits which occasionally billeted themselves on ordinary people.

Much of the time, of course, the ramblings of a man possessed must have

9

been hard to follow; much of the time, hardly worth following. Yet this did not necessarily detract from their influence. What mattered to the tribe was not whether a medium's voices made sense, but whether what they said could be interpreted in such a way as would make sense. When it could, its power through suggestion might be decisive. In much the same way, the oracle at Delphi was later not renowned for its clarity; it was how individuals reacted to its comments that mattered (the same, incidentally, could be said about most horoscope readers in the newspapers today).

And again, it did not necessarily matter – so far as the patient was concerned – what the interpretation was, provided that the disorder from which he was suffering happened to be one of the wide range which was capable of being dealt with through suggestion. He might be told to fast, or to eat, and he might benefit from either prescription, provided that he felt confidence in its source.

Divination, however, was often an erratic aid to diagnosis; and suggestion, for all its therapeutic power, was more likely to get rid of the symptoms than to remove the causes of disease. It might 'cure' a man of arthritis temporarily; it was unlikely to prevent its recurrence. And against many of the disorders that afflicted primitive tribes, it can have been of little value. Dietary deficiencies and food poisoning were a common consequence of the loss of the old animal instinct about what to eat, and what not to eat; and although occasionally divination of a missing ingredient may have saved tribes, showing them what to add to their diet, suggestion alone would be powerless to stave off the effects of beri-beri – or whatever it might be. And against infectious disorders, and epidemics, its usefulness was marginal. What was really achieved by suggestion, too, came to be attributed to magic; and this removed the incentive to find and preserve rational therapeutic measures. But although primitive medicine made little progress towards more scientific attitudes, its record is not quite so feeble as medical historians have made it appear. Most of them have been interested only by the discovery that in many different parts of the world, neolithic man used the operation of trepanning – as many primitive tribes do to this day. The common assumption has been that it was used to treat the kind of headache which makes people say 'I felt my skull was going to burst'. Whatever its purpose, it seems sometimes to have worked, as the patients not infrequently recovered: some were later operated on again in the same way. But it is more likely that the object of trepanning was to release demons imprisoned in the skull, and anxious (or so it must have appeared) to get out; or that it was part of some magico-religious ritual, perhaps with no therapeutic purpose at all.

There is a better example of an ingenious therapeutic technique, developed in primitive times. In India, a certain species of termite makes its nest by stapling leaves; the workers use their jaws as pincers to bring the leaves together, and the leaves are then stitched to hold them in the required position. Observing this, some early genius had the idea of using the termites to join the skin over a wound – and rendered stitching unnecessary by cutting off their heads and leaving the pincers in to hold the edges of skin together.

Primitive man also used many useful first-aid measures. Most of the tribes that have been studied by anthropologists have employed poultices, bleeding, massage and baths: most have also used a range of drugs prepared from herbs. Sigerist listed opium, coca, cinchona, ephedrine, caffeine, cascara, digitalis, ipecacuanha, podophyllum, pyrethrum and squill as coming from primitive folk medicine; soon after his death rauwolfia, the plant from which the original tranquillisers were produced, could have been added to that list (so, perhaps, could penicillin; mould poultices were a common folk remedy). It is possible that further discoveries will eventually show that other early herbal remedies, long since disused, are valuable – though the herbs in common use among primitive tribes are not necessarily the same as those which were used by man in prehistoric times. The discontinuity of the primitive mind tends, as Garrison noted, to substitute *propter hoc* for *post hoc* at every opportunity. Anybody cured of an illness with a new herbal remedy was apt to attribute the cure to the remedy, though suggestion was really responsible. As a result, herbs of real value might fall into disuse, supplanted by impostors.

This process was accelerated by the rise of magic. Naturally it was in the medicine man's interest to make himself indispensable; and one easy way to do this was to insist that herbs, however valuable in themselves, were all the better for an incantation spoken by or over the patient. To patients, this may often have been justified – if the magic impressed them, it helped to make them better. But eventually this meant that patients began to have faith in the magic, rather than in the herb.

Eventually, the magic would cease to impress, tempting the medicine man either to fraud, or to more eccentric remedies – because the more weird the incantation, the more likely some patients were to feel that it must have magical properties. Often, too, medicine men were driven back on exploiting their power over the members of their tribe for no better reason than to preserve their supremacy; and the spread of religions accelerated this process. The essential advantage priests possessed over the medicine man was that they could call upon divine assistance – and, if necessary, divine sanctions, including the threat of vengeance in an after life. There was no hard and fast distinction; between the two lay a middle ground, occupied by practitioners who can best be described as sorcerers, regarding themselves as priests but practising magic. Once instilled, though, the notion of omnipotent gods, and of an after life, helped to drag medicine still further away from its moorings in instinct and in pragmatism.

The therapeutic skill of the medicine men, though, should not be despised. There was a time, Sigerist recalled, 'when anthropologists considered them swindlers and humbugs, who fooled the people with a few tricks for the sake of material gain. Today nobody doubts that they are sincere and believe in what they are doing – just as the patient does.' Early medicine must often have been far from being 'primitive' in the pejorative sense. Medicine men used many techniques and remedies whose value was later ignored or forgotten, and is only now coming to be appreciated.

3

EARLY CIVILISATIONS

China

THERE is no ascertainable point in time at which medicine ceased to be primitive; but sometimes the processes can be observed by which it became systematised. This did not necessarily improve the patient's prospects; often it simply meant the imposition of arbitrary patterns of diagnosis and treatment based on mistaken assumptions about the nature of health and disease. The tendency of historians of medicine has been to concentrate on those systems which have come nearest to fulfilling modern requirements, to the exclusion of those explorations of what now appear to have been blind alleys. But this is surely a mistake – not simply because ideas which have been put forward in the past, but then rejected or forgotten, have so often later turned out to have been right (or, at least, to have pointed in the right direction) after all; but also because, whether right or wrong, some have exercised a lasting influence.

The most striking example of longevity in what the West has regarded as an eccentric system of medicine has been practised in China for over five thousand years: acupuncture. It can be traced back direct to primitive times; a form of acupuncture was practised in the Stone Age, and it has continued in China for at least five millennia without a break. In the rest of the world medical systems, like empires, have come and gone, so that above the folk-lore level there is no other direct link with early medicine.

Acupuncture had its origins in the 'Plus or Minus' assumption about disease; and it owes its survival to the fact that it fitted in with the Taoist philosophy which emerged in China, based on the belief that life is an interplay between two forces, Yang and Yin, light and dark, in perpetual contrast. In man, a balance between the two forces meant harmony, and that meant health; but if either Yang or Yin – Plus or Minus – became dominant, there

13

would be disharmony, and disease. In the treatment of disease, therefore, the concern was not with the symptoms, or the part of the body where they appeared. It was assumed that they *were* merely symptoms; a possible indication of what the trouble was, but otherwise not of significance. The acupuncturist no more thought of treating the symptoms than medicine men did; his object was to restore harmony by stimulating Yang (or Yin) so that the two forces resumed their proper balance. As soon as this was achieved, the symptoms would disappear.

As the system is practised today – and has been, for those thousands of years – acupuncture consists of sticking fine needles into the body to the depth of a few millimetres (just sufficient for them not to fall out) at predetermined points. For Stone Age man, the exact points may have been considered of little importance; acupuncture probably comes from the same stable as trepanning, the design simply being to release pent-up forces in the body. But the treatment must have worked: and out of it developed a system of puncturing, and the theory which rationalised it.

The theory assumed that the life force, compounded of Yang and Yin, flows through certain channels in the body; and these are related to points on the skin. From the nature of the symptoms, and also from taking the patient's pulse, the acupuncturist could ascertain which internal organ was involved, which channel was affected and which force was responsible. The needles were then inserted in the appropriate points, acting as a stimulus, or goad; Yang and Yin were restored to harmony, and the patient to health.

The undoubted antiquity of acupuncture has not been enough to enable it to command the attention of Western scientists; but recently it has enjoyed a surge of popularity in some European countries, and there have been other indications that the method deserves reappraisal. It has been demonstrated that the acupuncture points so carefully marked out on ancient Chinese charts were not just arbitrarily selected: they actually correspond to places where the skin has a different 'tone', which can be detected with the aid of a machine designed to indicate small changes of electrical resistance on the skin (the 'lie detector' works on much the same principle, though it is concerned to measure general changes in that resistance, set up by an individual's nervous reaction to questioning).

Acupuncture was not the only orthodoxy in China. Herbalism reached an advanced state of development there, as the Emperor Shen Nung's Herbal

Pen Tsao, published nearly five thousand years ago, reveals. If legend is correct, Shen Nung was an assiduous researcher in person: he is reputed to have tasted 70 varieties of poison in a single day. Many of the drugs he listed are still in use; and a few drugs in the herbal which went out of use in the course of time have been reinstated – ephedrine was derived from one of them.

Still, the chief interest in Chinese medicine lies in acupuncture; and the chief significance of acupuncture, it may well be, will be found to lie not in the points of the needles, but in the method of diagnosis by the pulse. Sir William Osler sensed this: in his *Evolution of Modern Medicine* he recalled how diagnosis had developed in China until the whole practice of medicine centred around its basic idea 'that each part and organ had its own proper pulse, and just as in a stringed instrument each chord has its own tone, so in the human body, if the pulse were in harmony, it meant health: if there was discord, it meant disease'. If this theory is correct pulse diagnosis has far greater possibilities than its limited use by Western doctors, who have mainly been concerned with rates and irregularities, would suggest – a view which the few Western doctors who have adopted it, confirm. Whether the average Western doctor would be capable of making effective use of the technique is another matter: at least one who took the trouble to try to master it – Colonel M. H. Shah – came to the conclusion that few Westerners now possess the necessary delicacy of touch.

Babylon

Of the other systems which evolved from primitive medicine, the best recorded is that which was practised by the Sumerians in Mesopotamia five thousand years ago; carried on there by the Babylonians and Assyrians; and adopted by the ancient Egyptians. This was sorcery systematised: health and disease, it was assumed, were cosmic phenomena, related to the condition of the universe (much as some arthritic people relate their pains to the weather). Religion, magic, learning, and science were all accepted as if within a spectrum, with the natural at one end and the supernatural at the other; a philosophy which the practice of medicine reflected.

First, the nature of the disorder had to be 'placed' in the spectrum; and for this purpose a seer, or diviner, would be invoked. According to his pronouncement, patients might take one of two courses. They might go to an

exorcist, who would prescribe the rites needed to drive out a demon, or pro-
pitiate an indignant god. Or, if the illness was deemed to have come from
natural causes, they could consult a general practitioner, who would undertake treatment with the help of elementary surgery or with drugs – the Babylonian *materia medica*, like all such lists dating from primitive times, exploited
herbs and other natural resources extensively; some of the drugs have remained in common use to this day (though since the discovery of antibiotics
and other newcomers, they are no longer so often prescribed).

That Babylon had something resembling a medical profession, in the
modern sense, can be gauged from the celebrated Code of Hammurabi, promulgated over four thousand years ago; the oldest extant professional rule
book. Its provisions have often been quoted: they indicate a higher regard for
the safety of the citizen than for the peace of mind of the practitioner:

if a physician shall make a severe wound with a bronze operating knife on the
slave of a free man and kill him, he shall replace the slave with another slave.
If a physician shall make a severe wound with an operating knife and kill him
. . . his hands shall be cut off.

Public health regulations were also strict, extending to intervention into private life where it was felt that individual laxity might harm the community.

Laws are a notoriously untrustworthy source of information about customs. They are revealing more of what the authorities want to be done than
what is actually being done; edicts imposing standards can often be taken as
a sign those standards are not being maintained. Nevertheless, the Code indicates that medicine had already, by 2000 BC, taken on a form and an organisation not dissimilar to that which we know today. How, then, to account for
the evidence archaeologists have presented that Babylonian medicine, so far
from developing along sensible empirical lines and progressing from the
irrational to the rational end of the spectrum, actually moved the opposite
way; so that the tablets belonging to the library of King Assurbanipal of
Assyria, dating from the middle of the seventh century BC, are infested with
demons, divination by omens, astrology, exorcism and incantations?

The evidence of those tablets, admittedly, is fragmentary; they have presented chronological difficulties to scholars, who have not found it easy to
date them with certainty. But it happens that the same process can be observed in ancient Egyptian medicine, about which we know a great deal

Opposite: Indian medicine man with sling and bow

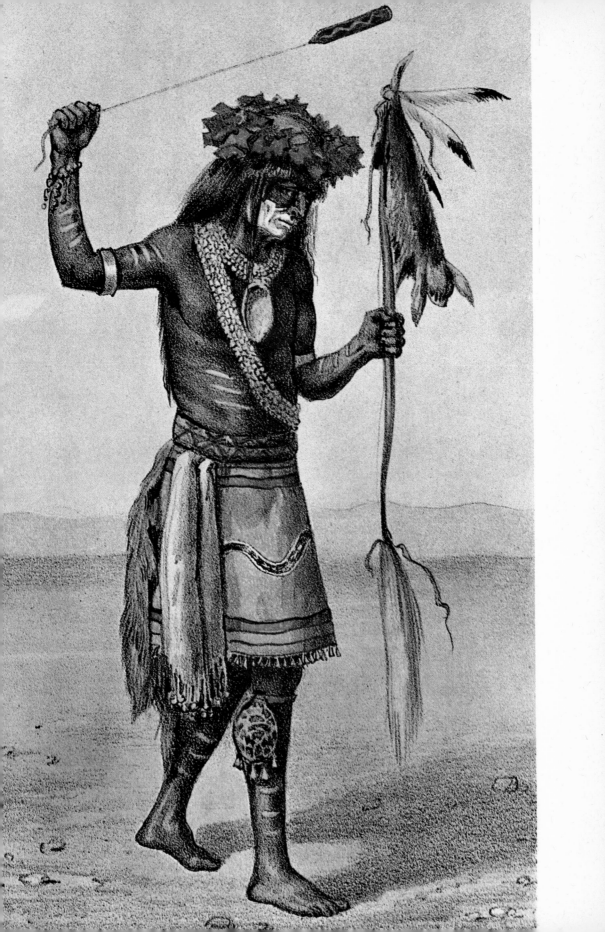

more – so much so, that Singer could misguidedly assert 'the history of medicine begins in that strange land whose very existence depended on the rise and fall of the Nile'. It would have been more accurate to say that the documentation of medical history begins there – at least as far as Western medicine is concerned. Papyri (scrolls) have been preserved, setting out medical notions and methods in some detail. The Egyptian custom of embalming the dead, too, has provided an unusual opportunity to investigate what kind of disorders people suffered from then (very much the same as we do now, apparently). The bones of the dead, which is all that remain from most past civilisations, are less revealing.

Egypt

The Egyptians, like the Babylonians, believed that health and disease were related to events in the cosmos; in the sun and the stars, which were identified with gods. Like the Babylonians they had their diviners; if a disorder was revealed to be at or near the natural end of the spectrum, it would be treated with natural remedies; tonics, emetics, enemas and so on. Honey, beer, oil, garlic and herbs were prescribed; so were certain drugs – opium, hartshorn and a few mineral derivatives, made up in the form of draughts, pills, or suppositories. The value of sound diet and of hygiene was recognised, and to some extent enforced on the public and on members of the profession.

The diviner, though, might decide that the disorder lay at the supernatural end of the spectrum; in which case the sorcerer was visited, and the treatment consisted of incantations, spells and other magico-religious rites. These formulae were designed to engage the sympathy or divert the wrath of the gods: Thoth, Isis, Imhotep and the rest. Again, it might be expected that as understanding grew of the nature of disease – and as new and more effective remedies gradually replaced old ones found wanting, filling gaps in the *materia medica* – practitioners and their patients would gain confidence in the remedies themselves, and begin to dispense with the incantations until the magic element either disappeared altogether, or receded into a formality, like grace before a school meal. In fact, the reverse happened. The ancient Egyptians in the early stages of their civilisation displayed a surprisingly extensive knowledge of anatomy, pharmacy and pathology; and their techniques, so far as can be ascertained, were basically rational, with relatively little reliance on magic. But, as Paul Ghaliounghi found from his researches, 'the classification of papyri according to the degree of archaism of their language has revealed the disquieting paradox that the papyri whose originals appear oldest are the most devoid of magic, whereas the more recent ones have gradually peeled off their medical polish, and kept only the superstition'.

This was to happen over and over again in the history of medicine. Quite abruptly, pragmatic modes of medicine would emerge, which for all their limitations appear by modern standards eminently sensible, and which should have provided an excellent opportunity for a rational therapeutic system to develop. But the current would flow relentlessly the other way; rationality would be overlaid with systematisation, or mumbo jumbo. Why?

There appear to be two main reasons; the first being that it is an inevitable tendency of any group of men practising medicine, whether priests, sorcerers, medicine men or physicians, to form a closed corporation and begin to develop a closed corporative mind. Such groups are under powerful pressures, for the sake both of their prestige and of their pocket, to make themselves indispensable. Any Egyptian schoolboy, presumably, knew that castor oil was a purgative; there was consequently no point in bothering the sorcerer if a purgative was all that was needed. But if it was accepted that any drug, to work properly, should have a spell attached, then the sorcerer's services would be required. And as he considered himself, a priest of the gods, to be a superior personage, he did not like his rights to be infringed by outsiders – or even by general practitioners; his attitude to them was probably very much the same as most doctors is today to chiropractors. Even if he did not consciously try to squeeze the general practitioners out of business, he would do his best to persuade patients that it was always wise to consult their sorcerer, just in case.

And sorcery, paradoxically, could be more effective. To begin with, it was better attuned to the culture of the times. Magic was not then, as it later became, something esoteric and rather disreputable: it was accepted in much the same way as Christianity is by the devout, as part of the general scheme of things, not to be challenged. In the present day, when belief in a deity has dwindled to the point when even those who consider themselves believers do not ordinarily think of their god as intervening directly to cause or cure an illness, we find it a little hard to put ourselves in the place of an Egyptian in the time of the Pharaohs; but for him the gods were real. Even the worldly wise, in all probability, had the imminence of cosmic forces so firmly implanted that they could not rid themselves of it – much as people to this day who do not consider themselves superstitious are nevertheless careful to throw spilt salt over their shoulders, and to say 'touch wood'.

In those circumstances, the power of suggestion must have been strong, whereas rational medicine was at a relatively rudimentary stage. The Egyptian *materia medica*, though it contained many useful remedies, was erratic; and the drift to sorcery under the Pharaohs probably did not involve the loss of many valuable aids or techniques. Nonetheless, Ghaliounghi's verdict that this drift was 'disquieting', is justified, because sorcery tended to decay into trickery – a process to be observed so many times in medical history that it is worth trying to account for.

The priest or magician who practised medicine has always (though he has not as a rule been aware of it) been subjected to pressures pushing him towards charlatanism. As suggestion played so important a part, it was inevitable that he should realise that patients who were impressed were also receptive. And, being gullible, they tended to be impressed by a man who appeared to have unusual – or better still, supernatural – powers. A sorcerer, therefore, who wanted to build up a good practice was always being tempted to reinforce his magic with conjuring tricks. When he was good at them, his patients would be impressed. If they were impressed, they stood a better chance of recovery. If they recovered, they would tell their friends, which would attract patients from a rival sorcerer – and he in turn would be tempted to resort to conjuring.

There is no need to assume, though, that the Egyptian sorcerers deliberately engaged in fraud. It is not, after all, considered fraudulent for a hypnotist to use some aid – a soporific formula, a flashing light – to put his patients into a trance. The kind of sorcery that the word 'Abracadabra' brings to mind, with its rituals and incantations, was not necessarily any more harmful – so long as it was used for this purpose. Where medicine began to go astray in ancient Egypt, as so often in other lands, was in the growing assumption that such aids were valuable not simply *as* aids, but in their own right; so that incantations originally designed merely to put patients into the right mood came to be regarded as having intrinsic healing powers – much as prayers, originally designed to help members of a Church to attain communion with their God, have so often degenerated into exercises in rote or even into penances, like the writing out of 'lines' at school. Amulets, too, began to be considered as having a therapeutic power of their own: any trinket, if suitably infused with 'luck', could be thought of as having an inherent capacity to ward off disease or accident – as they can to this day: there are no statistics of the number of people who carry a 'lucky' charm in which they have faith, at least to the extent of feeling worried if they mislay it; but it is probably surprisingly high. And eventually this weakens the power of sorcery, because it becomes too diffused – and cheapened. The sorcerer's temptation is not simply to use charms, but to sell them to patients, and the charms eventually fall into contempt – just as the relics of saints, sold by the Church, were to do in late medieval times.

In such circumstances, sorcery is invariably forced back on ingenious and desperate expedients to keep its hold; and this happened in ancient Egypt. It was no longer enough to lubricate a drug with a simple spell: the spell had to be recited a specific number of times, if it was to be effective: and it had to be recited with absolute precision. In this way a sorcerer whose prescription failed could put the blame on the patient, for not keeping to the letter of the instructions.

Presumably it was for the same reason that drugs, too, grew less rational, more esoteric. The general practitioner must have resisted the encroachments of the priest into his territory; and one way he could do so was by attributing remarkable powers to his own latest medicament. Obviously it could not be a herb or 'simple' which the patient knew, and could find for himself; the temptation was to prescribe compounds that became ever more complex and bizarre. Possibly the ancient Egyptians shared what was recently a common belief that medicine to be effective should be nasty; some of their drugs were of a nastiness unparalleled. Pig bile was prescribed for eye trouble, crocodile dung to prevent conception. The faeces and urine of animals or birds were particularly sought after and big-game hunters must have been the grateful beneficiaries – one remedy for baldness required equal parts of the fats from a lion, a hippopotamus, a crocodile, a goose, a snake, and an ibis.

It is just possible that some of the eye-of-newt, toe-of-frog remedies did not actually require newts' eyes or frogs' toes: the Egyptians may have named some of their drugs as the English named some flowers (snapdragon) or the Spanish, some wines (Bulls' blood). To take such names literally could be as misleading as it would for a historian of posterity to assume that a prescription for 'Purple Hearts' was taken literally by the twentieth-century chemist. But there must have been many grotesque remedies – as well as strange theories designed to lend occult potency to drugs; for example the notion of 'signatures' or 'similars'. The sorcerers of ancient Egypt were attracted by the idea that they should look out for similarity between, say, an affected organ and the remedy – as if nature was perpetrating ingenious puns: thus, a plant with a flower or a root shaped like an ear would be prescribed for earache, or a yellow plant for jaundice. To a people in whom the idea of the cosmos was strongly implanted, this did not seem ludicrous; it was just the kind of arrangement that beneficent gods would have made.

Degeneration of this kind in medical practice is usually closely related to a decline of a national culture: and so it was in Egypt. It was probably connected with the gradual falling off in regard for the gods: where a community loses faith in its traditional religion, its members are often tempted by eccentric beliefs – as if desperate for fresh certainties. The Egyptian gods, for all their influence, lacked stamina. One of the Pharaohs, Aknahton, was actually able to abolish them and proclaim a single deity, the sun god (and incidentally to secure a small niche in medical history; he had himself and his delectable wife Nefertiti portrayed holding their daughters up naked to the sun's rays, thereby qualifying himself as the patron of heliotherapy). On Aknahton's death the old gods were brought back, but they did not recover their influence over the community: and the expedients by which their priests tried to shore up their waning power grew even more effete. Eccentricities began to proliferate; and from having been highly regarded – Homer extolled it – Egyptian medicine fell into disrepute – a contempt reflected in the prophet Jeremiah's sneer when prescribing balm of Gilead to the virgin of Egypt: 'in vain shalt thou use many medicines, for thou shalt be cured.' Herodotus described Egypt as overrun with specialists, each insisting on their exclusive rights to some part of the body – another characteristic symptom of decline.

4

GREECE AND ROME

Aesculapius

At first sight, Ancient Greece appears to provide a refutation of the thesis that the craft of medicine suffers from a variation of Gresham's Law, bad treatment driving out good – or, rather, irrational driving out rational. The glimpses Homer gives of medical practice in the *Iliad* and the *Odyssey* suggest that it was then archaic by comparison with the Hippocratic era, a few centuries later; Homer's concept of health and disease was not very different from the Babylonians', except that as his gods were less remote, less consideration was given to the cosmos; diseases were directly attributed to the whims of individual deities. But there are indications that the attitude of the Greeks to medicine became less rational. Homer wrote of Aesculapius as a mortal: a pupil, admittedly, of the centaur Chiron, but obviously only one of many, and one whose main distinction was that he happened to be the father of two of the doctors in the Greek army. Yet four centuries later, Aesculapius had become a god, and an important one: Socrates' last recorded utterance as the hemlock took hold on him was to remind Crito that they owed a cock to him.

Aesculapius, legend asserted, had been only too successful during his mortal life. He had cured so many people, Pluto had complained, that Hades was becoming depopulated; and Zeus had agreed to remove him with a thunderbolt. Aesculapius was therefore deified, and temples sprang up where the sick could come to worship, and to seek for cures (some of the temples had been there before, but if they were attached to the Aesculapian cult, the deification raised their status). The temples were usually in secluded places to which the sick would come as on pilgrimages; on arrival they would undergo purification rites, before being conducted to a couch in the inner precincts for the night. There, it was assumed, they would be visited by the god, or one of his children, or perhaps a trusted emissary, such as a snake; and provided that the god was satisfied with them, their illnesses could be cured.

The cult of Aesculapius spread rapidly. Previously there had been only a second rank goddess of health, Hygeia; she was gradually eased still further down in the order of precedence, coming to be accepted as Aesculapius's wife, and later as one of his daughters (along with Panacea) leaving Aesculapius's supremacy unchallenged. His cult was helped by the fact that it fulfilled an economic as well as a spiritual need; treatment cost nothing, though patients who could afford it were expected to contribute to the cost of running the temples. At its peak, the cult probably represented the most successful attempt in history to fuse religion, magic and nature cure – diet, rest, massage, and hydrotherapy – into the service of healing.

Essentially, though, the Aesculapian method relied on suggestion. Sigerist, cited Lourdes as the nearest parallel; whoever has visited Lourdes, he felt, 'can well imagine in what frame of mind the Greek patient was when the great moment, long anticipated with hope and awe, had arrived, when he was going to face his living god. In such moments of greatest nervous tension miracles do occur, or at least happenings which are difficult to explain.' And, as with Lourdes, surviving case histories from Aesculapian sources suggest that the commonest cures were of people suffering from what would now be categorised clinically as hysteria – dumbness, deafness, or blindness caused by some emotional trauma. Of the rest, sufferers from stress disorders – headaches, sleeplessness, indigestion – must also have been good subjects for the treatment.

But as the years passed, the standards of the temples deteriorated; and, as with Egyptian medicine, it is easy to see why. The temples required funds for their maintenance; and the most successful in attracting wealthy benefactors were naturally those which could claim the most spectacular cures. If, as accounts strongly suggest, the therapeutic techniques sometimes approximated to present-day hypnotherapy, it is not surprising that spectacular cures – or at least remissions – were obtained; but hypnosis was not understood sufficiently well for its use to be put on a systematic basis, and the results must have been patchy. When a customer did not have a vision of Aesculapius, the priests of the cult were tempted to send in one of their number dressed as the god (or even to let loose a tame snake) to remedy that deficiency. This, at

23

least, was the accusation that was levelled against these establishments; and it would be surprising if it had no foundation. The priests would not regard their action as fraudulent in intent – any more than the artificial liquefaction of the blood of certain saints on their 'day' is regarded as fraud by the priests of the Catholic Church: they argue that it is a legitimate device to preserve the faith of the ignorant, who might otherwise be tempted away from the Church, at the peril of their immortal souls. The priests of Aesculapius would have had an even simpler justification: if the method cured – why not?

But the temples also came under pressure to provide medicine; and soon, drugs were being used in them. Wootton in his *Chronicles of Pharmacy* remarked on the increasing importance of drugs after the Hippocratic era, in the fifth century BC; it must have been related, he felt, to the new commerce with Africa and the Middle East. It was also related, though, to the struggles between rival medical factions. Naturally, the merchant wanted to sell his goods; it was as much in his interest that they should get the reputation of being wonder drugs as it is in the interest of the present-day pharmaceutical manufacturer. So, word was spread around to doctors who were not members of the cult, and from them to their patients, how successful the new drugs were. Rather than risk losing custom, the Temples began also to provide them, no doubt reinforcing them with such excuses as that 'the recipe came from Aesculapius himself'.

For a time this may have been effective; but it led inevitably to a falling-off in respect for the cult. The temples continued to flourish under the Roman empire, but they were not destined to exert much influence on the later course of medical history – except insofar as they might be considered as forerunners of Lourdes and other Church healing centres, or of modern nature cure establishments, which represent a secular version of the temple method.

Hippocrates

Until quite recently, Hippocrates was by far the greatest name in medicine; and to this day to refer to a historical figure as the Hippocrates of his time, or of his country, is the highest praise. He was born on the island of Cos around 460 BC, and consequently practised in the age of Pericles; the assumption has long been that as he did for medicine very much what Socrates did for thought – liberating it from its adolescence and encouraging it to become

Egypt

Hesy-ré, 'Chief of the Dental Physicians', an Egyptian court doctor of the third dynasty. Detail of a wooden panel from his tomb at Saqqâra

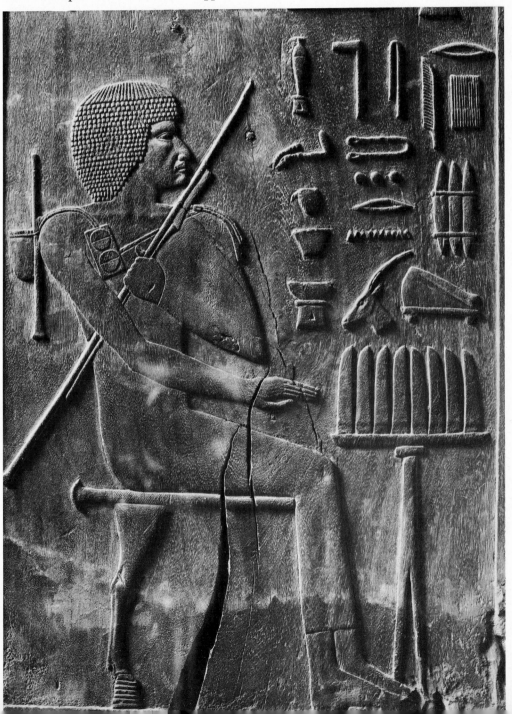

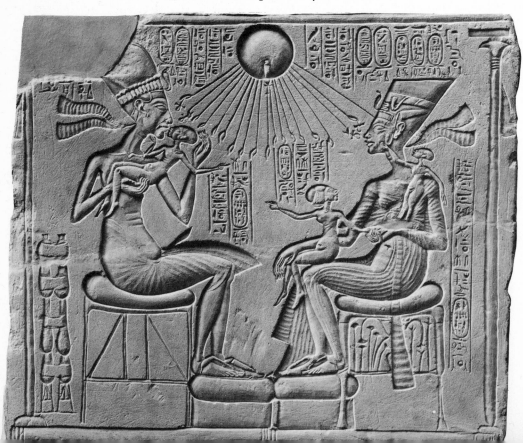

The Ebers papyrus, an Egyptian medical work of the sixteenth century BC. The text gives recipes prepared by the deities Nut and Isis for Ra, to cure his headaches

Aknahton and Nefertiti holding their children up to the rays of the sun

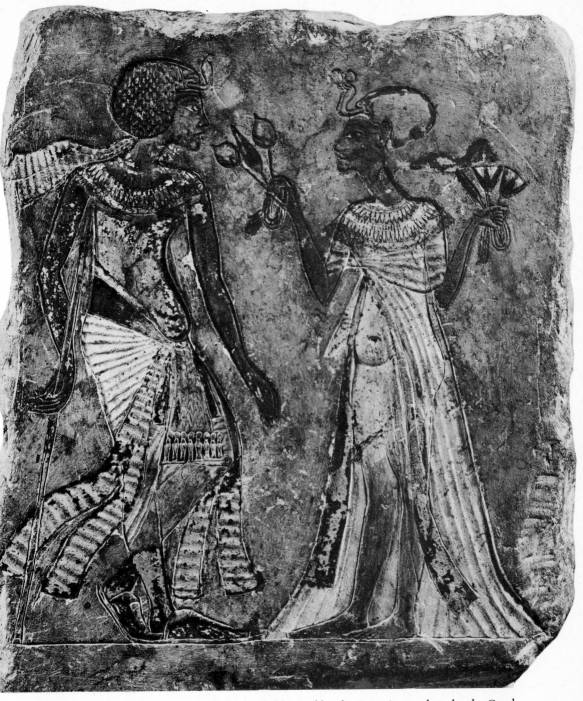

Nefertiti offering Aknahton mandrake, probably used by the Egyptians, as later by the Greeks, to induce sleep

Greece

Figures from a Bacchic procession. The frenzied dance of the bacchantes, like the later tarantella, had a therapeutic effect

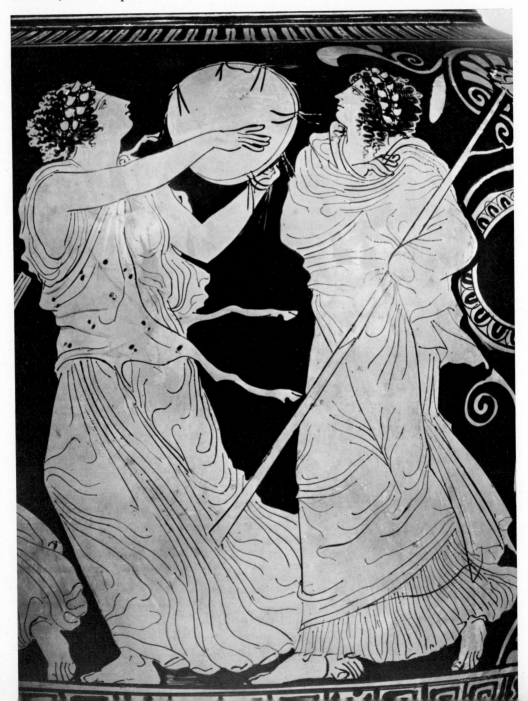

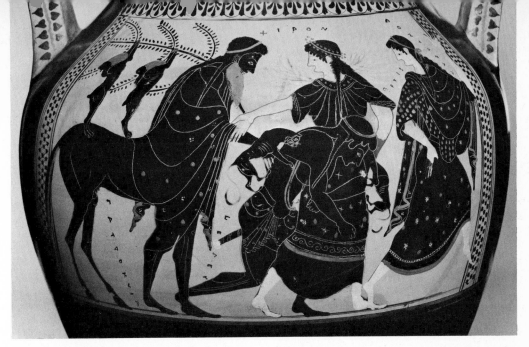

Chiron the centaur, famous in Greek mythology for his medical knowledge, giving assistance
to Peleus in his pursuit of Thetis

Patient in an Aesculapian temple licked by a snake while he sleeps, watched by an attendant.
He dreams that he is being cured by the God (scene on left)

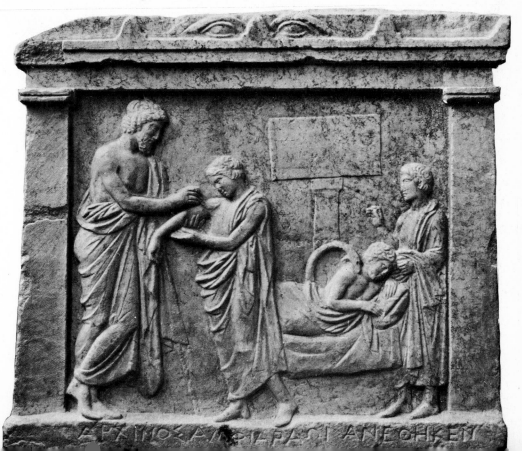

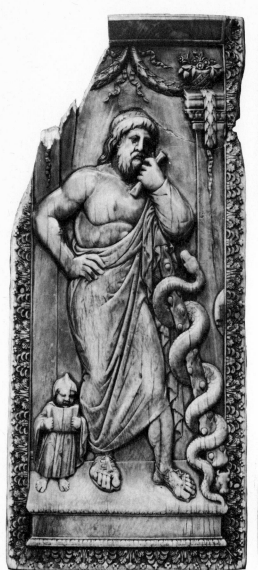
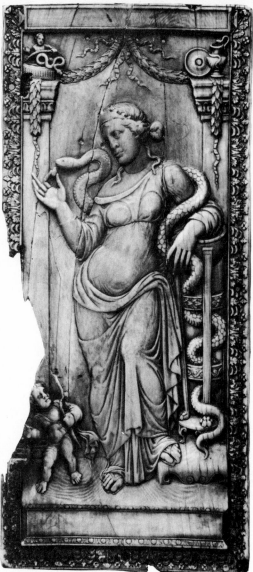

Aesculapius and Hygeia, presiding deities of Greek medicine, from an ivory diptych of *c.* 400 AD

Right: Hippocrates, from a Byzantine manuscript, holding in his hand a book with the most famous of his aphorisms: 'Life is short, the art is long'

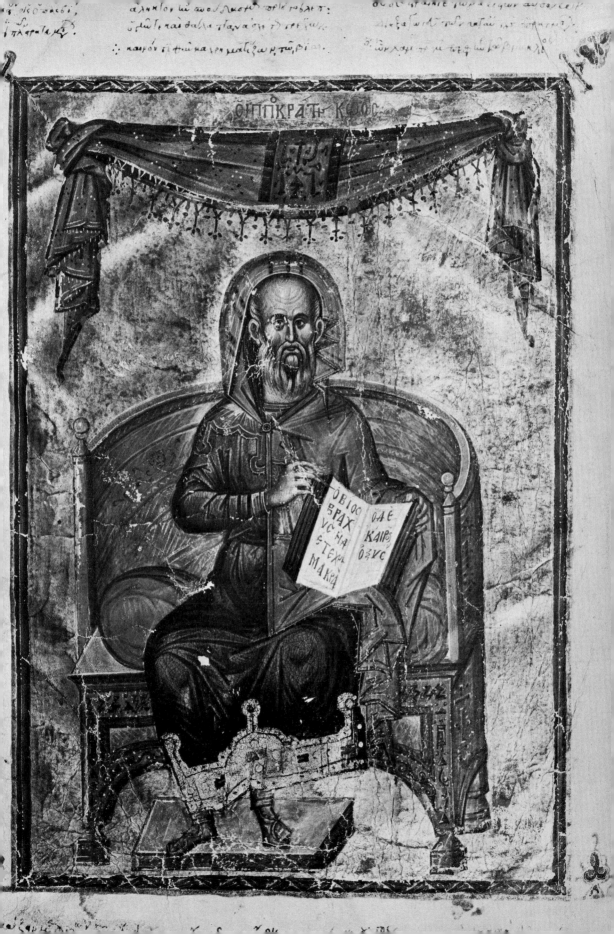

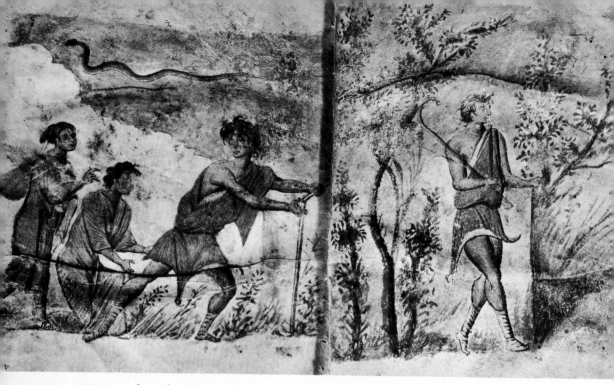

Miniature from the *Theriaca* of Nicandor, a Greek pharmacologist. The study of herbs and poisons was one of the most important fields of Greek medicine

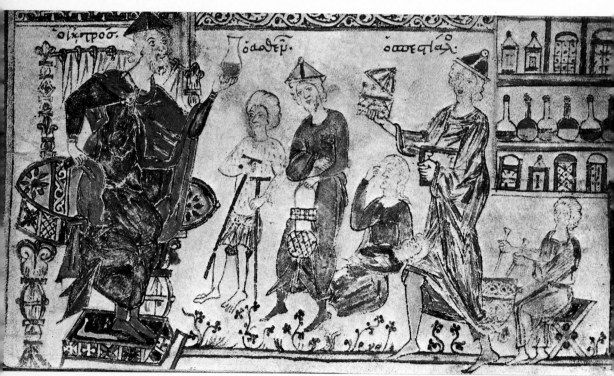

Miniature from a fourteenth-century Byzantine pharmacopeia showing a doctor examining urine, patients and an apothecary's shop

rational – he was eminently worthy to rank alongside his great contemporaries. He alone (it was believed) had been responsible for taking Greek medicine by the scruff of the neck, shaking out the magico-religious accretions, insisting on the observation and accurate recording of case histories, and, by comparing them, making possible the first systematic differentiation of diseases – as well as setting up standards for doctors (the Hippocratic Oath) of a kind that are still admired and accepted today. 'All that a man of genius could do for internal medicine,' Garrison claimed, 'with no other instrument of precision than his own open mind and keen senses, he accomplished ... to him medicine owes the art of clinical inspection and observation, and he is, above all, the examplar of that flexible, well-poised attitude of mind, ever on the look-out for sources of error, which is the very essence of the scientific spirit.'

But this enthusiasm, though revealing about the influence of Hippocrates on later generations, has had to be modified. Very little is known of Hippocrates himself. He is mentioned a couple of times by Plato, and clearly was well known as a medical teacher; but his name did not begin to bulk large until centuries later. And the works which used to be taken as by his hand have now been shown to be simply a collection of treatises by many doctors holding very diverse opinions – the collected contents, as it might be, of a small medical library.

Hippocrates is the classic example of fame attaching itself to an individual because he happened to be in the right place at the right time. Although not deified like Aesculapius – because as a rationalist, he was on the wrong side of the tracks – he was hero-worshipped. Yet there is no certainty that he even wrote one of the Hippocratic writings; and the only one which the evidence points to as his – because it fits in with the earliest description of his theories from an outside source – is generally regarded as one of the least convincing.

Medical historians have been understandably reluctant to let their hero slip out of their grasp. Even Sigerist, though he could not blind himself to the flimsiness of the evidence, continued to believe that Hippocrates himself had written some of the books (he had no idea which); and although he emphasised the need for caution before accepting later traditions about Hippocrates, 'legendary as they probably are', he excused himself for examining them in some detail on the ground that 'most legends contain an element of truth'. They do: but the 'truth' is much more likely to be about the people who related and embroidered them, than about their subject-matter – as many a later example has shown. Hippocrates appears to have been a man to whom later generations attached their anecdotes, beliefs and prejudices in very much the same way (though on a smaller scale) as the early Christians did to Jesus; traditions which reveal much less about Jesus than about the early Christians.

From posterity's viewpoint this is disappointing; but the slenderness of the evidence about Hippocrates himself does not detract from the significance of the Hippocratic writings – it merely demands a different way of looking at them. Their value, in a sense, lies in their inconsistency. They have been all things to all inquirers; almost every branch of medicine (other than those which followed the rival magico-religious line) has been able to trace its origins back to them; osteopathy and homeopathy vie with orthodox medicine to comfort themselves in the respectability of friendly references 'by Hippocrates'.

The reason that so many apparently diverse groups can feel at home with Hippocrates is that the writings are more concerned to observe and describe than to comment and criticise. They do not preach; they do not, as so many later textbooks have done, put forward a therapeutic system as if it were the only possible way of treating patients, ignoring all others. In fact they hardly concern themselves with this aspect of illness: their attention is centred on diagnosis and prognosis.

Perhaps the best known of the clinical descriptions is of the moribund patient; 'nose sharp, eyes hollow, temples sunken, ears cold and contracted and their lobes turned out, the skin about the face dry, tense and parched, the colour of the face as a whole being yellow or black, livid or lead coloured'. The kind of changes to be observed in the face of a dying patient were painstakingly noted; when 'the eyelids or lips or nose be contracted, livid or pale, one may know for certain that death is close at hand. It is also a fatal symptom when the lips are loose, hanging, cold and very white.'

But this – though it vastly impressed posterity, as the earliest known attempt at accurate observation from the bedside – was of little use to the patient. That doctors should be able to distinguish what was the matter with him, and what effect it was going to have, was of little benefit unless it enabled them to prescribe treatments of a kind that would cure him. And on treatment, the Hippocratic writings had little to say, above the first-aid level. Obviously the authors knew how to deal with the consequences of accidents, dislocations, fractures, and wounds; but on disease, all they ordinarily had to offer to the sick patient was rest and diet. The drugs they mentioned were mainly of the kind that would now be off-prescription: simple purgatives and emetics. So limited were the powers of these Hippocratic physicians actually to intervene to change the course of an illness that Asclepiades, three centuries later, could reasonably complain that so far as he was concerned, the Hippocratic observational method was little better than 'a meditation upon death'.

Yet the meditation is undeniably agreeable. The Hippocratic aphorisms are particularly endearing, with their air of refined melancholy: a couple of them have become household phrases – which, rather surprisingly, is unusual for medical dicta: 'desperate diseases require desperate remedies' and 'life is short, and the art (or craft) long'. It continues:

> ... the occasion fleeting; experience fallacious; judgement difficult. The physician must not only be prepared to do what is right himself, but also to secure the co-operation of the patient, the nurses and the auxiliaries.

The aphorisms are common-sensical, full of Socratic enjoinders to preserve the golden mean: to eat, drink or sleep either too little or too much is bad, and so on.

But the writings have probably owed their reputation chiefly to the delight they gave to those members of the medical profession who have wanted to escape from what they felt to be the stranglehold of religion and magic. Nineteenth-century rationalism, in particular, could look back to Hippocrates as its patron; and when, with the discovery of germs, the cause of disease had at last been found, holding out the prospects of finding rational cures, Hippocrates seemed to be finally vindicated. He himself had declined to propose cures, it could be argued, out of a proper sense of his limitations – realising it would have been futile for him to do so, as he did not know the causes of disease; and at least his patients had escaped the miseries and agonies from treatment based on false suppositions of the nature of illness – the bleedings and cuppings.

There is some truth in this. Lacking any positive theory of treatment, Hippocrates (for convenience, his authorship may be conceded) placed his reliance on the *vis medicatrix naturae*. In its pure form, this might be described as a belief that if the patient's life force is strong enough, he is going to re-cover: if it is not, he is going to die; so doctors should leave it up to his life force, merely removing impediments to recovery (for example, insisting that the patient rests) and giving his body every assistance (such as providing a suitable diet).

Had this theory been generally accepted, later death rates from disease would arguably have been much lower than they actually were, because fewer patients would have died from the effects of ill-conceived treat-ments and poisonous drugs. To this extent, the Hippocratic system of treatment was both rational and effective. But there was one insuperable objection to it: it required a rational community in which to *be* effective. And ordinarily, people are not rational about illness. Few patients trust their own life force implicitly; most want to see or feel that something is being done for them, when they are ill; the doctor who prescribes a treatment or a drug is, other things being equal, the doctor they will call in, rather than the man who simply tells them what they are suffering from, and how long they can expect to suffer. And in this, though patients may be foolish – in terms of un-necessary money spent, and unnecessary suffering undergone – they are not necessarily being unreasonable. If an illness is to be regarded as a temporary breakdown in the life force, then why not employ some device to do the life force's work for it until it has recovered? The doctor who promises to pro-vide a drug which will do just that has naturally been more popular with patients than more Hippocratically orientated colleagues.

For all the limitations and inconsistencies of the writings, however, Hippocrates deserves an eminent, if not a pre-eminent, place in medical hagiology; particularly for his emphasis on the importance of the doctor/ patient relationship. The rational strain – for example, the insistence upon the need to consider epilepsy not as 'sacred', but as no more nor less hu-man than any other disorder – did not lead, as it was later to do, into the barren materialism which ignores the patient, and thinks only in terms of the disease. As the nineteenth-century historian Edward Theodore Withington – old-fashioned in his approach, but perceptive – put it,

no one ever had a higher sense of the dignity of medicine; none showed greater respect for his patients; he even warns his pupils against exposing them unnecessarily during examination or whilst operating. The great object of the physician should be to benefit his patient, or at least do him no harm ... The wishes, and even the whims of the patient are to be indulged as far as possible, and a physician should rather lose his fee than trouble a sick person about it, for the memory of a good deed is better than a temporary advantage. He should also neglect no opportunity of serving the poor and the stranger, for 'where the love of art is, there is the love of man'.

The Systematists

There is no reason to suppose that Hippocratic ideas had much impact on medical practice at the time. The main rivals to the Aesculapian cult were not Hippocratic in any meaningful sense; for want of a better word they must be classed as Pythagorean.

The career of Pythagoras himself is so encrusted with legend that it is impossible to disentangle fact from fiction; but it appears that around 530 BC he left Greece for southern Italy to set up a religious-philosophic Order which was eventually to exert a profound influence on medicine. This philosophy arose out of an understandable dissatisfaction with the waywardness of the Greek gods, who were credited with behaviour more like spoiled and temperamental children than deities, driving the Pythagoreans not to agnosticism or monotheism but to a new and more austere conception of the cosmos, in terms of mathematics – 'a key to the riddle of the universe, and an instrument for the purification of the soul'.

The philosophy had some direct repercussions on treatment. Illness which could be regarded as emotional or mental was treated with music – mathematics expressing itself in sound: patients were goaded to a frenzy with the help of an orchestra, and then encouraged to fall into a deep trance-like sleep – a method, Arthur Koestler has suggested, which can be regarded as 'the ancestral version of shock treatment and abreaction psychotherapy'. But more important for the future of medicine was the preoccupation with mathematical balance, leading to a fascination with individual numbers – in particular the number four. It seemed to provide a simple and yet satisfying explanation of man's relationship to the cosmos through the balance of his 'humors' – body fluids: an idea which was to be dominant in medicine, under various guises, for two thousand years.

The humoral theory appears to have originated in India, an elaboration of the Yang/Yin hypothesis. There were three basic fluids, it was originally assumed – air, bile, and phlegm: air being cold, dry, light; bile being hot, fluid, sharp; phlegm being cold, oily, heavy. When the three were in their correct proportions, the body was healthy; when the body was not healthy, therefore, the cause must lie in an excess or deficiency of one of the humors. 'Wind' suggested an excess of air: to remedy it, oil was prescribed, being hot, oily and heavy, counteracting the influence of the air.

Whether the Greeks borrowed this and other ideas from India, or evolved them separately, has exercised scholars for centuries; Indian medicine presents such insuperable problems of chronology that the issue remains undecided, because of this it is impossible to evaluate with any confidence even the work of the Indian Hippocrates, Susruta. But whatever its origins, the humoral theory represented a brilliant intuitive guess at the significance of the bodily fluids. The trouble was that the humoralists could not agree among themselves *which* fluids were significant. Some Indian writers added blood to the original trio: the Greeks relegated air to a secondary status, and divided bile into two humors, yellow and black. It has been surmised that black bile was included because of the dark appearance of vomit and faeces in certain serious illnesses: but if it had not been observed, another humor would certainly have had to be found in order to preserve the Pythagorean symmetry, and to fit in with other contemporary quartets – such as the theory of Empedocles, a contemporary of Hippocrates, who asserted that there were four elements, earth, water, fire and air – to which the four humors could be linked. With sundry Yang/Yin style additions – hot and cold, wet and dry – it was possible to construct an impressive looking diagram to express the human condition.

Thus presented, the humoral concept looks contrived; but its basis – the idea of health as an equilibrium maintained by body fluids; illness, a symptom of balance disturbed – was eventually to be given formal sanction over two thousand years later. Where the Pythagoreans – using the term to mean those who thought in their terms – went astray was in trying to read too much into the theory. Naturally they hoped that it would give them a clue to treatment. Suppose, for example, that a patient was sweating: a look at the chart indicated that this must be related to his blood condition: could it be that this was an indication for bleeding? Excited by the possibilities, the Pythagoreans rejected Hippocratic ways, and set out to try to find, understand and exploit a therapeutic system based on the humors – a system, they

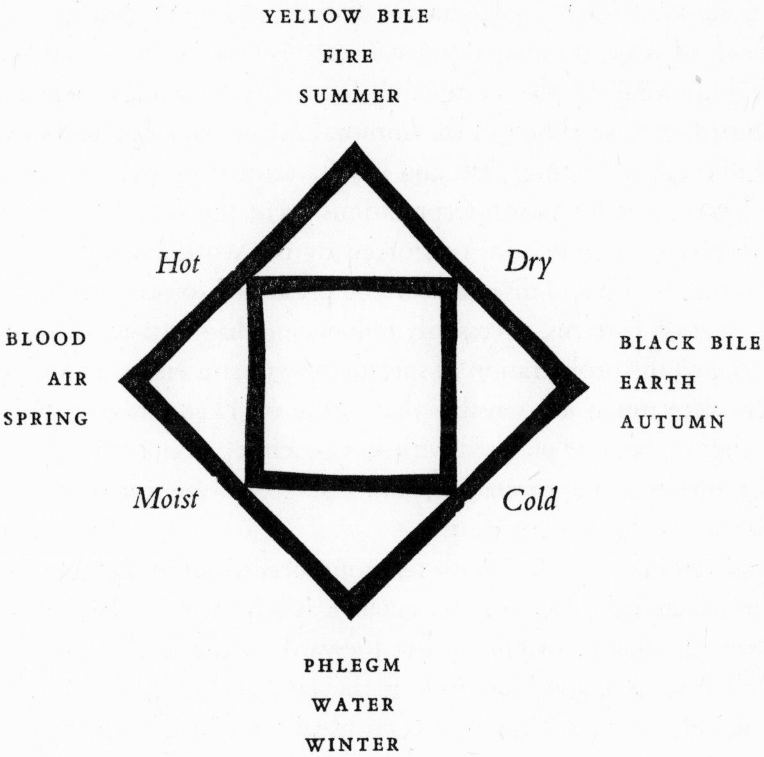

YELLOW BILE

FIRE

SUMMER

Hot   Dry

BLOOD   BLACK BILE

AIR   EARTH

SPRING   AUTUMN

Moist   Cold

PHLEGM

WATER

WINTER

felt sure, that must exist, in the same sense that the musical scale had existed before any human being had played an instrument.

Some of the efforts to explain the system were ingenious, the best known of them being the idea put forward by Aristotle's pupil Theophrastus in the fourth century, that the humors might be related to personality traits. People whose bodies were dominated by black bile, he thought, were melancholic in disposition. This in time was fitted into the theory, with sanguine, phlegmatic and choleric making up the required four; and as Sigerist – anxious as always to give credit where it was due – pointed out, several modern psychosomatic studies, notably those of Kretschmer, have shown that 'most of these ancient constitutional types are not fictitious, not the result of a desire to systematise vague observations, but are very real, and may be described in scientific terms'.

The implications of this discovery might, in fact, have been striking, as they pointed to treatment based not on the nature or type of disease – at least,

31

not exclusively – but on the nature or type of patient. But by the time that the idea of constitutional types was establishing itself, it was only one of several humoral theories competing for attention and acceptance.

The inherent weakness in the humoral theory was that anybody could regard himself as a humoralist, and base treatment upon his interpretation of the theory; but no two interpretations were the same. The nature of the Pythagorean doctrine, too, reinforced by the work and reputation of Aristotle – that health and disease could be presumed to obey certain immutable mathematical patterns, necessarily influencing diagnosis and treatment – later encouraged the proliferation of speculative systems embracing ideas many of which were much less sensible than those of Theophrastus; and medicine, like religion, became plagued with sects, each regarding itself as the possessor of the one true interpretation, and each requiring from its practitioners obedience to the one true faith.

It also meant – again, as with religious sects – that by the time an interpretation had settled down into acceptance as a doctrine, it had often diverged far from the theory originally put forward by the teacher to whom it was attributed: and a good example is the fate of Asclepiades, the friend and personal physician of Cicero, who is usually credited with the introduction of Greek medicine into Rome in the second century BC.

Asclepiades was irritated by what he felt was the excessive pretensions of the dogmatists – as they came to be known, though rationalists would be a fairer description: they regarded themselves as the true disciples of Hippocrates. He objected not simply to their negative 'meditation upon death' attitude, but also to the later humoral theory, because it seemed inadequate to him: and he put forward a counter-proposition which attributed disease to the condition not of the body's liquids – bile, blood, phlegm – but of its solids: illness came when they were too constricted, or too relaxed. This theory, also having obvious affinities with the Taoist Yang/Yin, greatly impressed some later students of the period; Albert Buck, for one, credited Asclepiades with almost visionary powers – far ahead of his time, in his grasp of the therapeutic importance of the notion put forward by Democritus that the body must be composed of atoms. And although the evidence about Asclepiades is too scanty for comfort, what little there is suggests that he was a reasonable man, not a crank: he is credited with an attempt to treat insanity with gentleness and sympathy; and although he

32

Opposite: Diagram of a pregnant woman, from a Persian anatomical manuscript

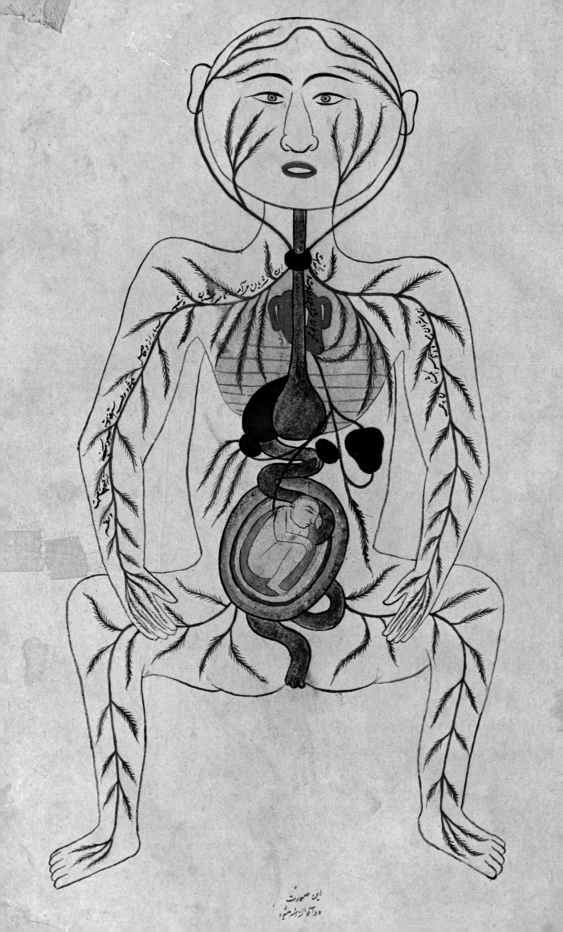

would have liked to intervene decisively to help the patient in illness, instead of relying on the patient's life force, he appears to have realised that few suitable means for such intervention were available (he advocated remedies not strikingly different from those recommended in the Hippocratic writings – diet, massage, hydrotherapy, and only sparing use of drugs). His followers, though, were attracted by the idea that illness was caused by the body's solids being either too constricted or too relaxed. This gave them the idea that treatment might be based on the principle of relaxing the body where it was restricted, and vice versa, which they held with such devotion that they became known as 'Methodics' or Methodists. And, as the obvious way to do this was with the help of drugs, drugs again began to find favour according to their success as constricters or relaxants. Out of their use in this connection another theory emerged that was to be of profound significance for the future of medicine: the doctrine of contraries, later to become known as allopathy.

The doctrine of contraries must have seemed, to those who encountered it, the logical extension of the humoral theory. This patient has a fever? Give him something that will restore the balance by cooling him down. That patient has constipation? Give him a laxative. Surely plain common sense! But there was a difficulty; to use contraries did not always accord with Hippocratic teachings about the importance of the life force. Suppose the symptom was not of a disease, but of the life force reacting to the threat of disease – as it did, for example, with vomiting, or with boils, both of them techniques that the life force had perfected to ward off its antagonists. In that case, the Hippocratic writings had indicated, the life force must be helped – if it could be helped at all – not by a contrary, but by something that would encourage the vomiting, or help to bring the boil to the surface, and to throw off the poison; a 'like' to cure a 'like'.

From this period it is possible to watch the ways diverge. Medicine divided into two camps; those who held to the doctrine of contraries (allopathy) and those who held to the doctrine of similars (homeopathy). To regard them as hostile camps is admittedly an oversimplification, because few doctors have subscribed exclusively to one doctrine or the other – the Hippocratic writings contain elements of both. But the division between the two, leading occasionally to violent discords, has remained important.

The chief centre of hostilities between the various sects which emerged out of the humoral theory was Alexandria, after its foundation in the fourth century BC. Here, for a while, the profession enjoyed a high reputation, resting chiefly on its members observing Hippocratic principles, notably in their respect for observation. Two names survive: Hierophilus, who is usually assumed to have been the earliest teacher publicly to dissect the human body (if he had not undertaken such dissections the knowledge of anatomy attributed to him was remarkable); and Erasistratus; but as none of their works survive, fact and myth about their careers cannot be separated, and most of the commentaries on them are based on their influence on the sects which grew up under them – or, rather, their inability to influence the course the sects took. Rejecting the humoral doctrines, Erasistratus had put forward the idea – to be echoed many times in later history – of the life force as a kind of airy, vital spirit, replenishing the veins: an intuitive appreciation of the role of oxygen. The chief cause of disease, he went on to assert, was a 'too much'; a plethora of blood in the veins, causing fever and other symptoms. Instead of adopting what must have seemed to be the commonsense course, and bleeding patients, Erasistratus rejected allopathy and used Hippocratic and homeopathic methods, mild and diluted medicines. But this did not prevent his disciples adopting allopathic methods; and the squabbles between them and the followers of Hierophilus eventually promoted a reaction towards empiricism – the rejection of all theories of medicine, and concentration on the patient and his symptoms. The idea was attractive to those doctors who were tired of wrangling about systems, and who felt that medical treatment should be based on lore, custom and experience. Why should it matter – their argument ran – that no theoretical reason had been adduced why a certain herb was effective in curing certain symptoms? Doctors should gratefully accept their good fortune that nature had made this provision, and not worry why. And of course if it were found that some form of treatment was not effective, it should be abandoned, however well-connected it happened to be – however well its accord with traditional notions about the humors, or their mathematical synthesis.

Hardly had the empirics established themselves, though, than they began to come in for some rough handling from their opponents, notably Galen, who felt that they degraded the profession to a folklore level, depriving it of the advantages of science (any form of medicine, as a contemporary historian has argued, 'lacking fundamental principles and approaching the bedside with a knife in one hand and a drug in the other, is striking in darkness'). But

the real trouble with the empirics was not so much that they rejected fundamental principles – in this they were wiser than rivals who accepted 'principles' uncritically – but that they did not realise the effect of the powers of
suggestion on the remedies they used.

The basic assumption of empiricism was that if a drug cured patients of
a certain disorder, then the drug must be effective. As they were unaware of
the extent to which its effectiveness lay in the doctor who administered it, and
his patients' faith in him, treatments began to proliferate which were apparently based on good empirical evidence, but actually based on suggestion.
Once again, the same kind of degeneration set in as had been observed in the
Egypt of the Pharaohs – and again, for the same reason. The doctor found his
patients more likely to respond to eccentric and grotesque remedies than to
the sensible and the ordinary. The name of one of the leaders of the empirics,
Serapion of Alexandria, is linked with such remedies as the specifics of the
camel's brain, hare's heart, crocodile's excrement, and wild boar's testicle.

Galen

What was required, clearly, was somebody who had sufficient erudition to
master all these diverse theories, and sufficient self-confidence to impose his
own pattern on them; and the mantle fell upon Galen.

Born in Pergamum around AD 130, Galen made a local reputation for himself as physician to the local gladiators before setting out in his middle thirties
in the hope of making an even bigger one in Rome. His ambition was quickly
fulfilled – mainly, if his own accounts are to be trusted, because of his remarkable diagnostic flair: he had the knack not simply of sensing what was
wrong with patients (which was not necessarily much help to them, if there
was no suitable remedy) but of sensing what would cure them. For some
reason – fear of catching the plague has been suggested; or, fear of the ani-
mosity of his rivals – he suddenly left while his reputation was at its peak, to
return to Pergamum. Not, though, for long; at the bidding of the Emperor
Marcus Aurelius, he set out again for Rome, where he was physician to five
emperors, spanning thirty years.

That he was persuaded to go back has been widely considered one of the
greatest misfortunes that medicine has ever suffered. To a surprising extent,
Rome had escaped the excesses of the various systematisers. Some commentators, admittedly, have felt that this detachment is no recommendation: 'the

original native Roman medical system', Charles Singer thought, 'was quite devoid of scientific elements and was that of a people of lower culture' – a deficiency not remedied until 'the entire external aspect of Roman medicine was changed by the advent of Greek science'. Such a proposition would have astonished and infuriated the elder Pliny, who took precisely the opposite view: for six hundred years, he claimed, Rome had got along fine without doctors, their absence having proved a boon to its citizens. Pliny's assumption was that the Romans were a healthy people because they paid scrupulous attention to hygiene, and had acquired an extensive knowledge of herbal remedies; provided that they made the right observances, they could expect to continue to enjoy the kindly protection of the gods: what more could they need? Certainly not doctors. There might be a place for medical auxiliaries – to give massage, say: but that was not a task for a free-born Roman. The fad (so Pliny thought it) for Greek medicine was both silly and degrading; and he quoted with approval what was perhaps the first of countless lapidary jests at the expense of the medical profession: 'he died by reason of the confusion of the doctors.'

This attitude was logical – Hippocratic, even; and Pliny's thesis, that Romans would have remained healthier if the Greek ideas had been excluded, is at least arguable. But by Pliny's time – the first century AD – medical practice in Rome had already begun to lose the simplicity he claimed for it. The evidence of his own writings reveals that the Roman medical catalogue was going the way of its predecessors elsewhere: it was a catalogue of rubbish, much of which Pliny accepted without even bothering to verify – though in many cases he could easily have done so: certainly he could have found whether radish placed on a scorpion would kill it, as the *Natural History* asserted. Besides, the herbs themselves were no longer considered efficacious without the assistance of magic. Pliny recommended a certain root for TB, but insisted that 'it must be dug up before dawn, and wrapped in wool taken from a sheep which has just had a ewe lamb'; 'some believe', he added, that 'the root should be dug up with a golden spade'.

The way magic had intruded into herbalism can also be seen in the work of Pliny's contemporary Dioscorides, who is usually accorded the title of the first European to compile a *materia medica* – as distinct from a botanical handbook. In the Hippocratic writings, for example, a certain five-leaved plant had been recommended for malaria. Dioscorides agreed, but with qualifications: three leaves should be taken by those who had 'tertian ague', but four by those whose fever recurred every fourth day; and in addition, he recommended the wearing of an amulet containing three crushed spiders.

The process of degeneration, then, was already well under way in Roman medicine; the growing reliance on pseudo-magic reflecting the decline of the Roman culture, as well as that falling off of faith in the gods which was later to give Christianity its opportunity. It also presented Galen with his. When he began to practise in Rome, doctors – from Greece and elsewhere – had already acquired some respectability; Julius Caesar had bestowed Roman citizenship on them, and Augustus exempted them from taxes for their efforts on his behalf. The Romans, too, uneasy with their own medicine, craved the promise of esoteric knowledge afforded by a foreigner; and Galen was the apotheosis of alien certitude.

Galen was well aware how to acquire a reputation: he adopted that air of bland self-confidence which is so much prized by patients longing for comfort, and all the more welcome to them if they happen to be emperors, used to command subservience. He left a description of the occasion of his successful conquest of Marcus Aurelius, which was to seal his reputation. The emperor had returned to Rome in triumph after a victorious campaign, and had feasted too well during the celebrations. Three doctors had been called in, taken his pulse, and prescribed drugs – with no result. Galen first roused the emperor's interest by declining to take his pulse, saying it was unnecessary, as there was no question of fever – the trouble was simply over-indulgence in indigestible victuals. With any other patient, Galen continued, he would have recommended wine sprinkled with pepper; but with kings, less drastic remedies were conventional, so he would simply recommend a poultice on the stomach – the emperor's usual, not very effective, remedy on such occasions. Marcus Aurelius sent for the poultice – but as soon as Galen had left, ordered wine, spiked it with pepper, and drank it, remarking that he was relieved at last to have a doctor with the courage of his convictions.

Apart from being so shrewd at the bedside, Galen was an assiduous anatomist; much of what he observed was accurate, and some of it perceptive; and the care with which he wrote up his findings made his work useful to teachers and, therefore, to students, anxious to show themselves proficient. As soon as his influence over Marcus Aurelius was established, then, Galen had every inducement to become arrogant and dogmatic; and he did.

No physician has aroused stronger feelings. He made little attempt to disguise his contempt for his rivals; and he stood rapt in contemplation of his own genius. 'I have done as much for medicine,' he was eventually to write, 'as Trajan did for the Roman empire ... I alone have indicated the true methods of treating diseases. Hippocrates, admittedly, led the way, but he did not follow it up: his works have grave limitations. He pointed the road: I made it.' And admirers have been inclined to accept him at his own valuation. To them Galen – even more than Hippocrates, a historical figure almost by courtesy – is the medical polymath: his service, as the American historian of medicine, A. H. Buck, put it, was 'to weld together into a single clearly written and easily intelligible system of medicine all that was good in the Hippocratic writings and in the disconnected, and at times antagonistic, teachings of the sects'.

Galen's system was indeed easily intelligible; but only by the use of distortions and over-simplifications to make everything fit. What he preached and practised was a mixture of personal experience and rival theories, all fused together into an impressive-looking but spurious Pythagorean structure. The actual remedies he recommended, apart from the fact that they required to be reinforced by magic, were often ludicrous; for although Galen did not invent polypharmacy, he revelled in it. 'It is the business of pharmacology,' he wrote, 'to combine drugs in such a manner ... as shall render them effective in combating or overcoming the conditions which exist in all the different diseases.' It followed that the way to decide on the best combination was to keep on experimenting and, whenever one of them worked, to apply it in future to cases of the same disorder. In this, Galen believed he was being empirical: he could not know how often a cure was effected not by the particular compound being tried, but by his personality. For all his arrogance, he seems to have remained unaware of the extent to which he, rather than his remedies, was responsible for his patients' recoveries. But although suggestion gave some striking results they were also inconsistent; the results given by his compounds were consequently erratic, too; and so they had to be 'improved' by experimenting with yet more drugs. In the end, a compound of a dozen or a score of drugs might be administered in a single dose.

It is possible to put up a defence of theory in medicine – as Scott Buchanan did – on theological grounds. If a community firmly believes that all creation serves some great final design, it is logical to search for the design, in the hope that when it is found, all mysteries will be cleared away, than to grub around empirically. But this requires a humility that few seekers after truth have possessed; certainly not Galen. The pattern, over and over again, has been for researchers to think they have grasped the design, and thenceforward to dedicate their careers to fitting all the evidence, Procrustes-fashion, to it.

To Galen's detractors, therefore, he appears a man who, for all his abilities, was a disastrous influence; particularly because he left his 'system' – 'a weird hodge-podge of nonsense, Aristotelian philosophy, Hippocratic dogma and shrewd clinical and experimental observations', as one of them calls it – to exert a stranglehold on the future: 'Hippocrates left medicine free, but Galen fettered it with hypotheses.' But to be fair to him, much of this criticism should be directed not so much at what he believed as at the rigidity with which his works were interpreted by his disciples. Had all his books been destroyed when his library was destroyed by fire in AD 192, his name would certainly now be held in respect, as a kind of Dr Johnson of medicine. But about a hundred of them survived, providing a comprehensive system of medicine on an apparently sound clinical basis. As with Hippocrates, too, the reader could be reasonably certain of finding in Galen's works whatever he sought in them; but with an additional assistance, which Hippocrates did not provide, that Galen actually boasted of his cures, and related them to the theory so ingeniously that they had the appearance of being an integral part of the cosmic design. It was relatively easy, therefore, for Christians or Moslems to accept and embrace Galenism – simply leaving out what did not fit, and insisting that what Galen had regarded as the life force came not from the cosmos, but from God, or from Allah. From this it was a short step to imposing dogmatic interpretations, laying down what could, and what could not be considered as medical orthodoxy – the Truth.

But though Galen was not himself responsible for squeezing medicine into this mould he cannot be exonerated entirely, because the temper of his mind, and therefore of his writings, was authoritarian. As a consequence, it was Galenism, rather than Roman medicine, that was to survive. Yet there had been some justice in Pliny's claims for his city, particularly in the field of public health. The measures that were taken to keep the city and its inhabitants clean were unsurpassed. The main sewage system was in operation as early as the sixth century BC; later, the aqueducts were built to provide the city with ample fresh water; public baths and facilities for exercise were provided not only in Rome but in outposts of the empire, for its defenders. One Roman hospital dating from the first century AD has been excavated in Germany; it anticipated the corridor design that was later to attract Florence Nightingale, and become for a while the conventional pattern.

But public health measures are early victims in times of civil upheaval of the kind Rome was so often to suffer in her decline; and they rarely survived onslaught and occupation by an invader. In any case, though the Romans did much to prevent disease, they did not master it; some authorities have suggested that it was to their failure to control malaria that the fall of Rome can ultimately be traced. In time the empire acquired a structure which made epidemics hard to avoid. The growth of cities around the empire, Zinsser argued, few of them enjoying Rome's hygienic facilities, and the improvement of communications between them and the rest of the world, was calculated to provide the raw material for plagues, and to spread them; 'a sample survey of the frequency, extent and violence of the pestilences to which Roman Europe and Asia were subjected, from the year one to the final Barbarian triumph, will convince the unprejudiced that these calamities must be interpolated in any appraisal of the causes that wore down the power of the greatest state the world has known.'

When – whether from epidemics, or political incompetence, or moral decay, or a mixture of these and other contributory causes – the Roman Empire finally disintegrated, its medical legacy to posterity was not its aqueducts or its hydrotherapeutic establishments, soon to crumble into elegant decay, but an elaborate system of alien medicine whose ideas and methods were a direct repudiation of those of Ancient Rome. And whatever the deficiencies of Galen's system, an admirer could claim, his 'colossal personality loomed up through the long night, as a brilliant guiding star to light the intricate pathways of medicine'. During that long night, systems of any kind were to be hard put to survive in Europe; but chance was to bring them to a place of relative safety, not far from where the Babylonians had cultivated their system, so that they could be maintained, and returned to Europe, more or less intact, when dawn broke.

Rome

Aeneas attended by his surgeon for a wound in the leg received on the battlefield. Fresco from Pompeii

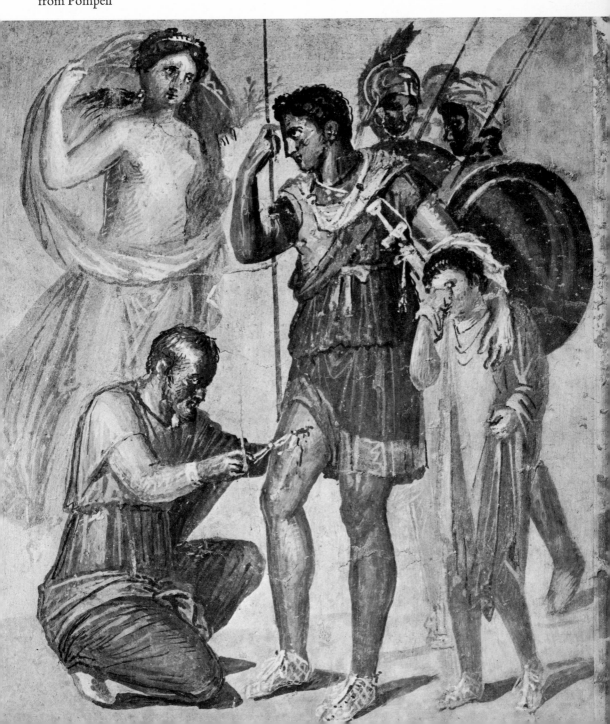

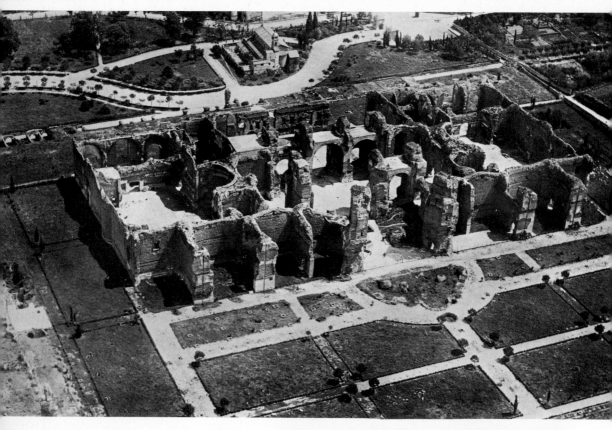

Baths of Caracalla built 206–17 AD, where 1,600 people could bathe. They were equipped with cold, warm and hot baths and gymnasiums

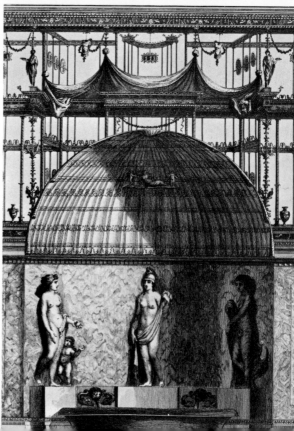

Detail of wall decoration from the Baths of Titus, showing the luxurious setting; from an eighteenth-century engraving

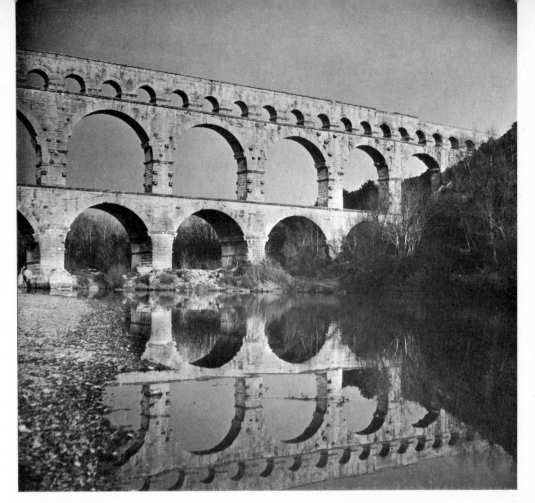

Pont du Gard near Nîmes, one of the finest Roman aqueducts. Roman systems of drainage and water-supply transformed standards of public health in the outlying provinces of the Empire

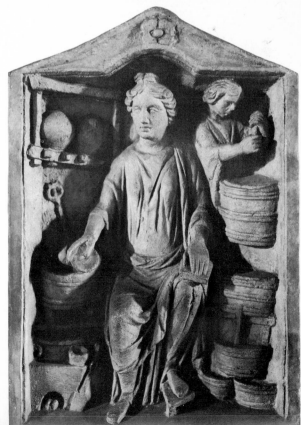

Apothecary's shop in Roman Gaul, showing that Roman medical influence was not confined to public health

Galen enthroned with some of his forebears in the field of pharmacology, the herbalists Crateuas, Dioscorides and Nicandor; Andreas, who was Ptolemy IV's personal doctor; and the Alexandrians Apollonius and Rufus

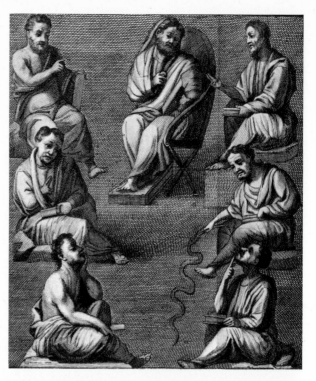

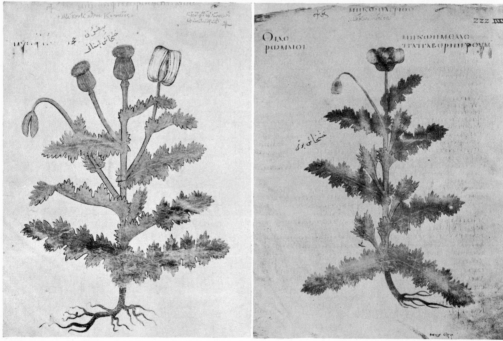

Two types of poppy from a sixth-century manuscript of Dioscorides' herbal, one of the many Greek works which were an important influence on Roman medicine. Poppies were long used for their narcotic and anaesthetic properties

Arab Medicine

Avicenna, from the lacquer binding of a Persian seventeenth-century edition of his *Canon*

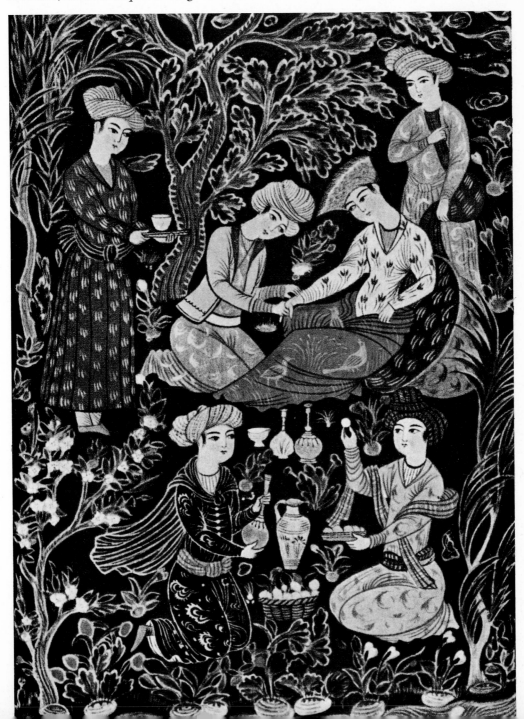

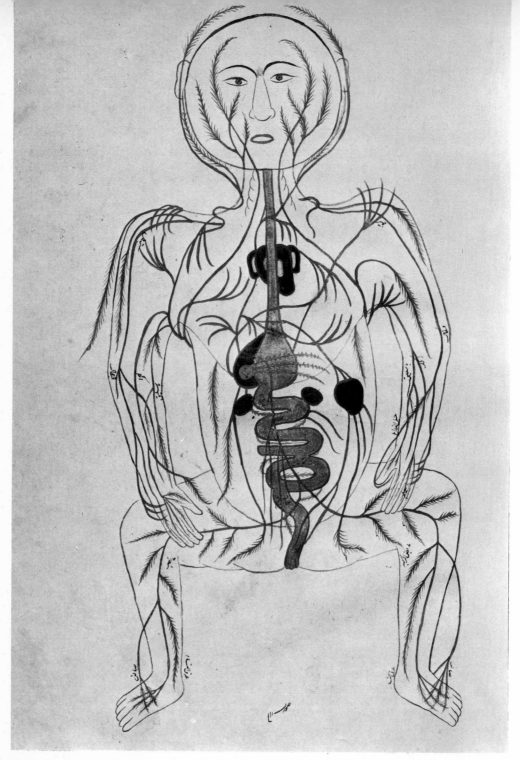

Persian diagram of the blood-system, believed to be derived from the anatomical studies of the Alexandrian medical schools

English thirteenth-century miniature of the blood-system, showing the indebtedness of European medieval medicine to the Arabs

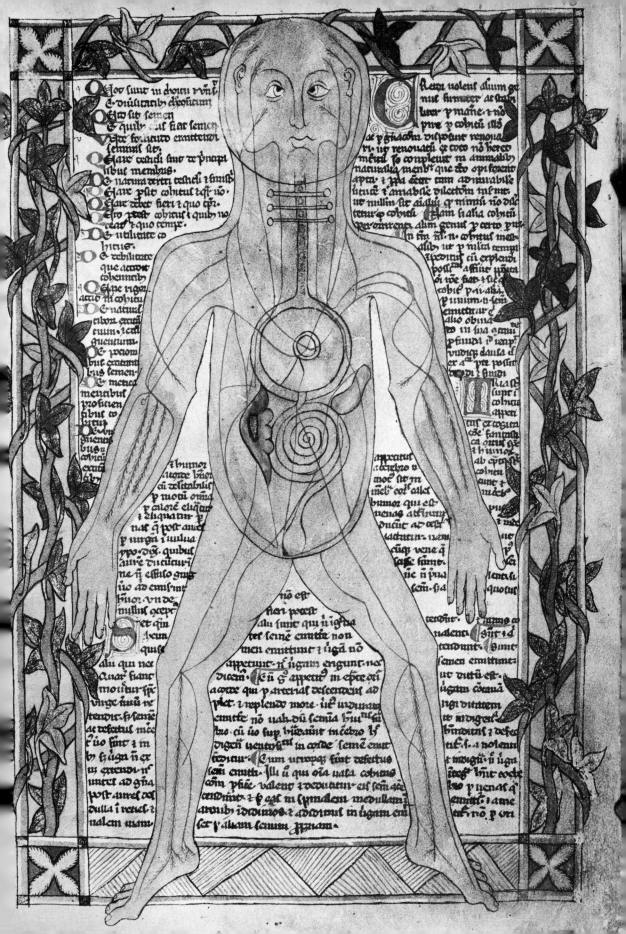

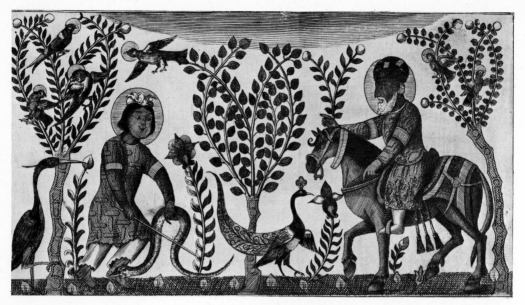

Miniature from an Arabic manuscript on Vipers and Theriac,
translated from a Greek
pharmacological work

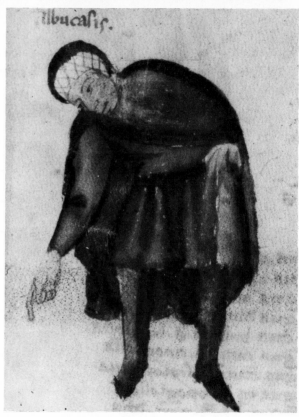

Albucasis the Spanish surgeon and
dentist stooping to inspect a
medicinal plant

5

ISLAM

Rhazes and Avicenna

ARABIAN medicine might never have impressed itself on posterity, except as a curiosity, had it not been for a bitter religious dispute in Byzantium in the fifth century AD. The protagonists were both unattractive: the crafty, cruel Cyril, Patriarch of Alexandria, and the hardly less disagreeable Bishop of Constantinople, Nestorius. Nestorius was worsted; having dedicated his life to the extirpation of heresy, making himself notorious for his savage persecution of the Arians, he found himself persecuted and proscribed as a heretic; and his followers, to avoid the Arians' fate, had to remove themselves out of reach of the Church's vengeance. They eventually settled in Persia, under the protection of Chosroes the Blessed. For want of an alternative livelihood, some of them exploited the knowledge of Greek they had brought with them, including medical lore from Galen and Hippocrates; and their knowledge and talents, coupled with those of other refugees and visitors – notably from Buddhist India – produced a fine ferment in the medical arts in and around Chosroes' amiable court.

Chosroes died in AD 579; half a century later Mohammed was established in Medina. By a second stroke of good fortune for Arabian medicine, although authoritarian by temperament he turned out to be tolerant of the diverse breeds of medicine that had flourished under Chosroes' wing. He happened to share the widespread contempt of his countrymen of that epoch for traditional Arabian medical lore; and the Koran has little to say on the subject. Because he had little interest in preserving the old ways, he was prepared to accept the new.

Inevitably, clinical traditions arose associated with him; the fourteenth-century Arab historian Ibn Khaldun could refer to them in terms of little respect. The Prophet's mission, he insisted, 'was to make known to us the prescriptions of the Divine Law, not to instruct us in medicine', and he cast doubt on the medical prescriptions handed down as 'authentic'. Sensibly, though, he did not dismiss them altogether: 'if one likes to employ these remedies with the object of earning the Divine Blessing, and if one takes them with sincere faith, one may derive from them great advantage, though they form no part of medicine properly so-called.' The dominant figures during this period were unorthodox – Rhazes and Avicenna; and stories about their skill, ingenuity and wit abound. Such legends inevitably attach themselves to whoever is the most celebrated doctor of his time. This is not, of course, exclusively a medical phenomenon; a certain type of club story still attaches itself to the name of Winston Churchill, in much the same way. But it is constantly found in medicine; and Rhazes – and still more, Avicenna – were early beneficiaries.

Rhazes, a Persian, born in AD 850, was for a time a musician; then a philosopher noted for his pungent heterodoxy. He became interested in medicine almost as a hobby, but eventually it absorbed him totally, until his spreading reputation led to his appointment as physician-in-chief to the hospital at Baghdad. Tradition has it that when he was consulted about the site for the hospital he hung up a carcase at each of the four corners of the city, and selected the corner where putrefaction had been slowest – revealing that the connection between putrefaction and disease was beginning to be recognised, if not understood. This may be legend – as, indeed, may be the 'hospital'; but Rhazes' reputation rests safely on his writings, many of which have survived. He was a careful observer, mapping diseases with such precision that his descriptions still excite admiration of clinicians; particularly his differentiation, for the first time, of the symptoms of smallpox from those of measles.

Rhazes was Hippocratic by conviction, and his aphorisms show the Greek influence; notably his insistence that remedies which sapped the strength of the patients should be avoided; his belief that symptoms which appear dangerous, like fever, are not necessarily so – they may be nature's expedient to cast the disease out; and his advice 'when you can cure by a regimen, (diet, rest, etc.), avoid having recourse to medicine; and when you can effect a cure by means of a simple medicine, avoid employing a compound one'. Above all, Rhazes emphasised the importance of the doctor/patient relationship: 'the healing art, as described in books, is far inferior to the practical experience of a skilful and thoughtful physician.'

Avicenna, born in 980, was destined to make an even greater mark. He was an infant prodigy, quickly acquiring the self-esteem that pervades his writings ('At twelve years of age I disputed in law and logic . . . medicine is no hard and thorny science, like mathematics and metaphysics, so I soon made great progress; I became an excellent doctor'). This did not make him popular with contemporaries, but patients were impressed. He was one of those men who appear to have the gift of ceaseless energy; days of writing followed nights of drinking and making love; and his *Canon* ranks in stature and influence with the works of Hippocrates and Galen. For the historian of Arab medicine, Professor Browne, (who thought Avicenna the equal of Aristotle), 'its systematic arrangement, its philosophic plan, perhaps even its dogmatism, combined with the immense reputation of its author in other fields beside medicine, raised it to a unique position in the medical literature of the Muslim world' – so that the earlier meritorious works, including those of Rhazes, 'were practically abrogated by it'. The *Canon* was to become a standard textbook in many European medical schools, where it held its place until the seventeenth century.

What is more interesting, though, than the hotch-potch of earlier ideas that the *Canon* represented was the early flowering of psychotherapy under the Caliphate. There had been intimations of it before in the Socratic dialogues, with their analytic technique; in case histories attributed to Erasistratus – by his disciples, and to Galen – by Galen; but Rhazes and Avicenna have a reasonable claim to be the first to utilise the method as standard therapeutic procedure.

Again, it is dangerous to give credence to individual cases, as Avicenna was incurably boastful; but the proliferation of his examples indicates his interest. A typical example concerned a woman at court with a postural defect which had deprived her of the use of her arms – and consequently of her usefulness at court. A doctor, called in, suddenly stripped her of her veil, which caused her to blush: then, he stooped down and lifted her skirt over her head. Hastily, she pulled it down – and realised that she *could* move her arms, after all. Avicenna attributed the cure to the blush 'dissolving the erring humor'; diagnosis by hindsight would suggest the woman's ailment was hysterical in origin. Whatever the reason, the shock treatment worked. This interest in the power of mind over body was not confined to Avicenna: other examples from this period were attributed to Rhazes, including one which has also been repeated in many different versions later.

An irascible Emir, who had been suffering from stiffening rheumatic joints, sent for him to loosen them. Rhazes tried the standard remedies of the time, with no success; then, as a last resort, pretended to threaten the Emir with a knife. The Emir sprang to his feet, to ward off the attack – and Rhazes explained that the provocation had been therapeutic.

But perhaps the most remarkable of the cures attributed to Avicenna was described by a twelfth-century Persian writer; his way of dealing with a case of insanity. He was called in to see if he could cure a prince, suffering from the delusion that he was a cow, who went around lowing, begging to be slaughtered and converted into beef. Avicenna sent word that he was coming in the capacity of a butcher; but on examining the 'cow' pronounced him too lean to be worth slaughtering; first, he must be fattened. The prince, delighted with the idea, began to eat – and gradually, as he regained his strength, the delusion disappeared. The story was often re-told by medical writers as a curiosity; but it was not until nearly a millennium later that Freudian psychoanalysts were to rediscover this technique of entering into a psychotic's fantasy life, in order to provide a bridge for him to return to reality. The process has been described by Robert Lindner in *The Fifty Minute Hour*, in the account of how he treated a research physicist who had begun to live in a science fiction world; and some psychotherapists feel that if the method can be perfected, it presents a new hope for the treatment of schizophrenia.

A fresh examination of the medical chemistry – alchemy – used by the Arabs might also be revealing. When Arab learning spread to Europe, this was one of the branches of medicine which aroused most interest; Rhazes, particularly, had done much research into it. Some of it was speculative, with the aim of transmuting baser metals into gold, but this was far from being the only objective. Useful chemical processes, such as distillation and sublimation, were perfected; the Arabs used their knowledge to carry out detailed investigations of drugs (the word 'drug' comes from the Arabic, as do many other standard scientific terms). Pharmacy emerged in the Caliphate as a speciality of its own: previously the physician had had to compound his own drugs, but now he was relieved of that task by specialists, as he is to this day.

Alchemy was later to become suspect in Europe, partly because of its links with sorcery, partly because some of its practitioners abused their skill for purposes of fraud. But there have recently been attempts to rehabilitate its reputation, notably by Louis Pauwels and Jacques Bergier in their *Le Matin des Magiciens*. The authors' contention is that a great deal of valuable research must have been done by alchemists, some of which could still be of value today if it could be rescued from the oblivion into which it has fallen. If they are correct, the possibility remains that Arabian medicine may yet emerge as significant in its own right, rather than as the largely fortuitous channel through which ancient Greek medicine was preserved for the West.

This may sound unduly optimistic, but it has to be remembered that there has been no systematic investigation of these sources: and that past researchers have often brought closed minds to their task. They have tended to be on the look-out for good, sensible, quasi-scientific descriptions of symptoms of a kind that might appear in a modern textbook, in order to present them as evidence that a Rhazes, say, was a man before his time. He was: but though the fact that he was able to make the first steps towards differentiating measles from smallpox is to his credit, it cannot have been of much help to his patients, for no treatment at that time was likely to benefit them either way. A fresh study of the writings might reveal much that was missed by earlier researchers.

Sometimes, after all, they missed even straightforward cases of discoveries made, and then forgotten until centuries later. In the thirteenth century, Ibn an Nafis deduced that the blood flowed from the right side of the heart to the left through the lungs: a remarkable deduction, considering that he was prevented by his faith from dissecting the human body – unless, of course, he merely claimed that his faith forbade him, in order to forestall rumours that he had engaged in dissection. But his work was not noticed until the 1930s.

Even the Arabian poets have something to offer the researchers. Browne quoted the tenth-century writer Al Mutanabbi, describing a fever with which he had been smitten, in terms which echo Rhazes' feelings. The fever is not likened to an enemy – to some hostile influence; but rather, to a vexatious mistress:

> And it is as though she who visits me were filled with modesty.
> For she does not pay her visits save under cover of darkness
> I freely offered her my linen and my pillows

45

But she refused them and spent the night in my bones
My skin is too contracted to contain both my breath and her
So she relaxes it with all sorts of sickness
When she leaves me, she washes me (with perspiration)
It is as though the morning had driven her away
And her lachrymal ducts and flooded in their four channels
I watch for her time (of arrival) without desire
Yet with the watchfulness of the eager lover
And she is ever faithful to her appointed time — but faithfulness is an evil
When it casts thee into grievous sufferings.

The Cordovans

Avicenna was the last of the great names in medicine to emerge in what are now regarded as the Arab countries, but the other extremity of what was then the Moslem empire, Spain, was still to introduce a few more: notably Albucasis. Albucasis stands out because of his interest in surgery, which elsewhere in the empire had been regarded by physicians as an inferior, not very reputable, pursuit – a stigma which surgeons were to have the utmost difficulty in shedding; to this day, in fact, Albucasis' main interest – dentistry – is not regarded as being quite on the level of medicine: not, certainly, by doctors.

Many of the innumerable ideas and gadgets linked with the name of Albucasis may have been attributed to him because he was the first to describe them in detail; but the fact that he was prepared to write a treatise on surgery at all was a measure of the intellectual freedom possible in Spain under the Moors, at that time. In the twelfth century there even seemed a possibility that Moorish medicine would come to rival in reputation that of Rhazes and Avicenna; Cordova, in particular, provided a remarkable centre of learning as well as of commerce. 'Where medieval Europe was darkened at sunset,' as one enthusiast described it, 'Cordova shone with public lamps; Europe was dirty, Cordova built a thousand baths; Europe was covered with vermin, Cordova changed its garments daily'; and with its fifty hospitals, not to mention its seventy public libraries, Cordova held out the same kind of attraction for the aspiring doctor as the court of Chosroes had once had, at the other end of the empire.

For a while, it appeared possible that even the great Galen might be toppled

from his pedestal. His supremacy was challenged by Avenzoar; and though
Avenzoar's name is linked with a clinical eccentricity, the bezoar stone – a
growth sometimes found in animals' stomachs, and for a while prized as a
therapeutic aid – he was by general account a careful observer and a skilful
doctor, prepared to back his own judgments against the traditionalists. His
pupil and friend Averroes promised to be still more remarkable. He began
as a student of law, becoming first a magistrate and then a provincial gover-
nor; but he preferred to regard himself as a philosopher and as a physician,
and in both, he won esteem for the freshness of his attitude. But this was to
be his undoing: it got him into trouble with Moslem fanatics when they
came into power, determined to end toleration of other religious groups.
Averroes was disgraced and imprisoned.

Jews were also persecuted. Some were given the choice between accepting Islam or banishment, and among those who judged it wise to leave
Cordova was Moses Maimonides, a merchant. He eventually reached Pales-
tine. The year – 1165 – was not promising for immigrants, who found themselves engulfed in the ferocious struggle between Christians and Moslems
for Jerusalem: Maimonides nearly lost his life as an apostate, and the family
business collapsed, compelling him to look around for a fresh source of income. He turned to medicine, and eventually, after some years of struggle,
was fortunate enough to find a protector in Saladin.

Of all the patrons of medicine in history, Saladin is one of the most attractive – tolerant even of Christians, in spite of the crusades, and in spite of
the memory of the massacres in which Christians had slain some tens of
thousands of Moslems in Jerusalem, and herded Jews into their synagogues in
order the more conveniently to burn them alive. Maimonides' luck turned;
in the 1170s he became the head of the Jewish community in Cairo, and
during the last part of his life he was its respected elder statesman. To judge
from those of his writings that have survived, he was Hippocratic by conviction, advising simplicity in medication along with plenty of fresh air and
close attention to diet. He also repudiated magic; and his aphorisms, though
tending to be platitudinous, are full of good sense. But his teachings had no
time to take root; when he died, early in the thirteenth century, the Moslem
empire was on the verge of collapse. Cordova fell in 1236: Baghdad in 1258;
and the influence of Arabian medicine was thenceforward to be felt not in
its own birthplaces, but in Europe, where Arab writings, and in particular

the *Canon* of Avicenna, were to continue to dominate medical teaching until the end of the sixteenth century.

The generally accepted verdict of Moslem medicine has been Meyerhoff's: it 'reflected the light of the Hellenic sun, when its day had fled, and shone like a moon in the Dark Ages. Some bright stars lent their own light, and the moon and stars alike faded at the dawn of the Renaissance, though their influence remains to this day.' Recently, though, there has been growing restiveness about this picture, as an over-simplification. But before assessing the significance of the Arabian medicine in the Renaissance period, it is necessary to look back at the medicine which was being practised in Europe in medieval times, to see why it acquired an unsympathetic image – and to judge whether it was deserved.

Albula in oculo

Surditas

Nasus incisus usq3 ad aures

Apostema retro aures

Macule faciei

Labia vlcerosa

Inuasio bene magnu i collo

Apostema sub brachio

Vulnus sicut plaga percussum

Inuasio aueb... oculi fa...

Iustus fetor

Struma in collo

Vuln... fra... gladii retro ce...

Vuln... ifud hui carnes in ... tu vtraq3

Ossa fracta vbicumq3

Inuasio stoa ventis

Splenius

Cor

Fel iecur

Splen

Iunctura magna

tra... ferio i gladii

Inuasio vene vbi quis cessat n...

hasta br...

Inuasio viscera magna

Apostema i membris

Vuln... penetratu ad vtraq3 ptes vtraq3

Inuasio vesice Ictaluo

Vuln... vi iugq3

Vuln... psunde fixuj vbiniq3 variole p totu corpus

Sagitta cuius ferru remãsit i carne

Vulnera humorosa

Vuln... fluxile vbiniq3

Vuln... augustu huj foramine vbini

Paralisis vtraq3

Inuasio ferri seu vtrin iu pede

Prurit p totu corpus

Venue vtraq3

6

THE MIDDLE AGES

Galenism

'A THOUSAND years of darkness' is a characteristic chapter heading to sum up the history of medicine after the fall of Rome; such judgments as 'Galen was the final star that shone in the twilight of antiquity, and when his effulgence was extinguished there settled over Europe a darkness that was not lifted for many centuries' abound. Accepting this conventional verdict, Charles Singer justified it on the ground that anatomical and physiological inquiry ceased absolutely on Galen's death: 'the curtain descends at once . . . the dark ages have begun. Rational medicine in the pagan world descends into darkness' . . . and so on.

This attitude was understandable. Lifting the curtain and letting in a little light presented formidable difficulties, owing to the comparative paucity of sources. But Singer's implication that medicine had been rational before the dark ages, and ceased to be during them, reflects the real reason why so little interest has been displayed in medieval medicine. Because it was dominated by religion and magic, it has been dismissed as unscientific even in aspiration, and therefore as unworthy of serious attention.

This attitude, which is still widespread, might be summarised thus. 'From the time of Hippocrates to the death of Galen theories of medicine proliferate. Some of them were eccentric, but at least they represented a groping towards a rational therapeutic structure based on more exact knowledge of the workings of the human body. But after Galen's death progress ceased, and medicine regressed into sorcery. Only at the Renaissance was progress resumed; only at the Renaissance, therefore, does medical history become significant once more. In the interim, admittedly, one or two bright stars shone out in the darkness – individuals like Alexander of Tralles, institutions like the

Opposite: 'Wound man', showing the various injuries that a medieval doctor might be called upon to treat

Salerno school: they deserve to be mentioned, though, not because they were representative of medical practice of this time, but because they transcended it. The practice itself is not worth bothering about.'

It is hard to believe that Sigerist would have accepted this convention, had he lived to write the projected volume of his history dealing with the Middle Ages. To him, the medicine of any period was revealing – not only about the community in which it was practised, but for posterity; because medicine strips off civilisation's mask. In an era when people pride themselves on being rational (as in the eighteenth century) when the rationality is really only intellect-deep, the popular medicine of the time will reflect the stresses and fears accumulating beneath the surface. In such circumstances, commonsense remedies cease to command confidence: esoteric and quack nostrums abound. It is easy to be patronising about this, and say that 'every country gets the medicine it deserves'; but it would be nearer the truth to say that every country gets the medicine it needs. If suggestion is the most potent single therapeutic force, it follows that the most potent medical systems and remedies will be those which best capture the public imagination. The wearing of a talisman – if it carried conviction – must often have been more effective, in medieval times, than any prescription from the available *materia medica*.

To speak of Galenism as rational, then, in contrast to medieval irrationality is misleading. Apart from its many built-in inconsistencies and inaccuracies, Galenism had one striking disadvantage: although authoritarian in design, it was so presented as actively to encourage different interpretations of the same symptoms. Empiricism – at least in its early stages – had tried to relate treatment to symptoms; but the Galenist doctor had to try to relate treatment to the state of his patients' humors; and, as he had no yardstick to judge what that state might be, there was scope for endless confusion.

That a few practitioners realised this can be judged from a complaint by Priscianus, a Byzantine doctor, in the early fifth century:

As the patient lies on his bed prostrated by the severity of the disease, there quickly comes into the room a crowd of us physicians. No feeling of sympathy for the sick man have we, nor do we realise how impotent we are in the presence of those forces of nature. Instead, we struggle to the best of our ability to obtain charge of the case; one depending for success on his powers of persuasion, a second on the strength of the arguments he is able to bring forward, a third on his readiness to agree with everything that is said, and the fourth on his skill in contradicting the opinions of everybody else. And as this quarrel goes on, the patient continues to lie there in a state of exhaustion. 'For shame!' nature seems to say, 'You men are an ungrateful lot! You do not even permit the patient to die quietly; you simply kill him!'

But a doctor who confessed these Hippocratic sentiments to his patients could soon expect to have no patients – as well as losing all his friends in his profession. So if he shared Priscianus's insight, he would be tempted to give patients what they wanted; at no small cost, sometimes, to his own peace of mind – as Alexander of Tralles, a sixth-century physician who eventually settled in Rome, came to realise. His bias was towards pragmatism, and he acquired some notoriety by daring to express sceptical opinions about Galen, and by insisting that the treatment ought to be guided by symptoms rather than by theories. Yet this very pragmatism led him to accept and prescribe such treatments as:

Procure a little bit of the dung of a wolf, preferably some which contains small bits of bone, and pack it in a tube which the patient may easily wear as an amulet.

Or:

For epilepsy take a nail of a wrecked ship, make it into a bracelet and set therein the bone of a stag's heart taken from its body whilst alive; put it on the left arm; you will be astonished at the result.

Alexander was aware that some of his prescriptions sounded ridiculous: he excused himself on the ground that patients, like besieged cities, must be defended by whatever means put heart into them; and that although there was no rational reason why amulets should do so, in fact they did. In time, he hazarded, a reason for their potency would be discovered.

Christianity

Galenism of this nature provided what may loosely be described as the orthodoxy of the Middle Ages; but it acquired a powerful competitor in a therapeutic system introduced into Europe from the Middle East. Although Babylonian medicine had virtually disappeared after the collapse of its civilisations, it had left an offshoot, practised by the Hebrews. And whereas in Babylon, as in Egypt, the distinction between magic and religion had remained blurred, for the Hebrews with their emerging monotheism the distinction became

51

significant. Their whole attitude to health changed, and with it, their methods of treatment.

A community which believed in magic regarded disease as a consequence of malevolence: the patient was the victim of somebody or something. A community which believed in religion thought of disease as a mark of divine displeasure; and where there was but one God, assumed to be just, disease must be the consequence of sin: the patient was his own victim. This made a different attitude to treatment inevitable. A medicine man could reasonably claim that he was going to effect a cure by employing counter-measures against the witch, or whatever it was causing the illness: but a priest could hardly claim to effect a cure by the employment of counter-measures against God.

The priest's medical functions, therefore, tended to be restricted. He might still be employed for purposes of divination, to ascertain why the gods were offended; but he was not asked to treat the disease in the way that sorcerers did. And it was logical that he should not be expected to prescribe drugs; any tribe or race which believed in the absolute power of their god over the lives of men would naturally tend to believe more in the efficacy of pleasing or placating that god – sacrifice, prayer, whatever it might be – than in medicaments.

This did not extend to everyday disorders; a man who caught a chill or had indigestion did not necessarily feel that he was being punished. Nor did it extend to preventive medicine; God, it was assumed, would expect that men should do their best to preserve their health by whatever measures recommended themselves to the community, for the same reason that he would expect them to feed, clothe and house their families. In their public health precautions the Hebrews went even further than Babylon: so far, in fact, that Garrison credited them with being the founders of prophylaxis, and described their priests as 'medical police'. The health regulations in the book of Leviticus contain much that would be approved by present-day sanitary authorities, especially the regulations about isolating patients with certain types of disorder, and disinfecting and fumigating their premises; the command that everybody must be allowed to have one day's rest a week could also be considered a valuable therapeutic innovation. But there are signs in Leviticus of the kind of neurosis that afflicts individuals who must continually wash their hands, as if to wash away their guilt. The Hebrews overdid it.

Yet this was understandable. Disease was not simply an affliction to them; it was a warning. Ordinarily it could be interpreted as an intimation of divine displeasure; but it could also be a sign that God was testing the faith of the victim – as he had done, according to the legend, with Job. And the Christian Jehovah, apart from being omnipotent and all-seeing, obeyed the strictest standards. He was, in fact, the embodiment of those standards; he could do no wrong, and he expected his chosen children to do no wrong, either. If they did, the Recording Angel was there to make a note of it; and where they persisted they could be sure that their wickedness would be punished with eternal damnation and hell fire.

In such circumstances, agonising tensions are bound to occur. Individuals are prompted by their instincts to do what comes naturally, but their consciences tell them it is sinful. These conflicts are bad enough when the individual is aware of them; much worse if, as so often must have been the case, they are repressed. In such circumstances, as Arthur Guirdham pointed out in his *A Theory of Disease*, mental derangements become common. The conscious mind, instead, of acting as friend and guide to the unconscious, has to spend all its time trying to stamp out its rebellions; the tensions mount, and eventually causes an explosion – a fit, or a psychotic interlude. Of such symptoms, the Bible gives abundant evidence.

The manifestations of disturbance were not always ugly. The take-over bids for control of the mind were sometimes made by forces which, though inexplicable (as they are to this day) were not manifestly malign; individuals or groups might suddenly find themselves in a trance with the gift of tongues – speaking a language they had never been taught. But often the form that the explosion of irrationality took appeared to lend confirmation to the belief that it was the work of the devil. The unconscious mind, when it expressed itself, could do so in terms very similar to those which, by convention, the devil used to mislead the susceptible. It is as if in communities where belief in devils is strong enough, it is exploited by the unconscious forces seeking to liberate themselves from the tyranny of conscience, and acts as spokesman for them; so that when the derangement comes, it manifests itself in the form of diabolic possession, with – apparently – the devil speaking through his victim's mouth.

Now that belief in Satan has gone out of fashion, this kind of disorder has become rare; and the tendency has consequently been to discount diabolic possession as an old wives' tale – mistaken diagnosis. But the people really were possessed – even if the devil was in their own imagination, a projection of their community's fantasies. The test of the quality of Hebrew medicine is not whether diabolic possession happened to be the correct scientific explanation of this very prevalent form of mental (and sometimes physical) disturbance, but whether it was a reasonable hypothesis, given the circumstances and ideas of the time; and, still more important, whether it held out possibilities for effective treatment.

It did: exorcism. Exorcism was the natural and probably often the only effective available remedy – except, occasionally, shock. In the contest for control over the victim's mind, exorcism represented the bringing-up of a powerful ally – belief in God – for the forces of conscience; provided that they had not already suffered too decisive a defeat, they could sometimes be rescued with its help. To be really effective, though, exorcism required the confidence of the people not simply in God, but in the priesthood as representatives of God. Where the reputation of the priesthood was low – as it was to become in Israel, largely for reasons that the word 'Pharisee' immediately bring to mind – their influence waned; and a new therapeutic method was needed which would serve the true believer. Jesus provided it – as well as providing a new concept of God, so that the Christian, believing himself entitled to mercy as well as justice, would be less likely to suffer from intolerable sensations of guilt.

Jesus was to exert more influence on the course of medicine than any other man before or since: far more than Hippocrates, or Galen, or Avicenna. This might have been true even if, like Mohammed, Jesus had had no interest in disease as such; if he had simply commended the sick to the attention of his followers – along with the poor, the meek, and the downtrodden – as in need of help: for in that case the Christian attitude to the sick would not have been so very different to the attitude that was actually to establish itself in the Middle Ages, and which remains with us, though in diluted form, to this day. But Jesus was deeply concerned with the sick – as the Essene sect had been. His healing mission, as it was to be called, was one of his constant preoccupations; he employed specific techniques which have interesting affinities with those of primitive medicine; and he set out to create a medical cult, by passing on his ideas to his disciples.

Yet it is possible to read the standard histories of medicine and remain hardly aware that Jesus existed, let alone that he was the founder of a system of medicine. Garrison, Singer, even Osler, did not so much as mention his name; and Guthrie, though crediting Israel with contributing to the progress of medical science by promoting a social conscience and by instituting measures for public health, nevertheless asserted that 'no great physician appeared among the Jews, nor indeed any medical men at all'.

The reasons for this silence are not difficult to appreciate. Jesus's assumptions about the nature of disease and his healing methods have gone out of fashion. This alone would not necessarily disqualify him from consideration; so, after all, have Galen's assumptions and methods; and this has not deterred historians from devoting a great deal of space to Galen on the reasonable ground that for fifteen hundred years his influence on medicine was very great. Yet although they have found it a simple matter to analyse Galen's teachings, criticising and deriding their inadequacies, they have shirked an assessment of Jesus's contribution. The reason is obvious. They have realised that they would have to be critical; to be so, they feel, would give offence: therefore they had better ignore the subject altogether.

Paradoxically, the more devoted Christian doctors are, the greater as a rule will be their reluctance to discuss the subject in print. No doubt Sigerist, with his embracing humanism, would have tackled it sympathetically, had he lived; but men who have been believers, or at least good churchgoers, throughout their lives are frequently among the most violently prejudiced against the use of Christian ('quack') healing methods, and the most contemptuous about claims for miraculous cures, from Lourdes or elsewhere – in spite of the fact that their scepticism, if carried to its logical conclusion, would involve them in believing that Jesus must have been either suffering from delusions, or a fraud.

Battle has been formally joined – by theologians rather more often than by members of the profession – only over Jesus's healing miracles: and this also helps to explain why serious consideration of Christian healing has been burked. Christians have always assumed – as they still do, though more warily – that God has reserved powers. The thunderbolt is a force of nature, but it can in certain circumstances be wielded by God to punish the wicked. Pneumonia, too, is a natural phenomenon, but it can be contracted through an act of God; and – still more important, now that the idea of God deliberately making people ill has become repugnant – recovery from it can be brought about by the faith of the victim, or through the efficacy of prayer. But to the great majority of doctors, even those who are Christians, this idea of supernatural intervention is repugnant. Healing miracles, they feel, are either legends or case histories capable of a natural explanation. And between these camps the possibility of rational discussion has been small, as both have believed fervently that there is no possible way, and never could be a way, of reconciling two incompatibles.

But just as such phenomena as witchcraft and voodoo can now be reconciled with scientific theory, so Jesus's healing prowess can be explained – and not just explained away, after the old rationalists' fashion. Jesus's thesis that there was a merciful God who, through his son, could restore health to the sick, was what the members of the Hebrew community in which he lived were craving for (except, of course, the Establishment: the Pharisees). And as many of the disorders prevalent at that time arose out of tensions resulting from the strictness of the community's code, they would have been particularly susceptible to treatment by the form of release which Jesus offered. The 'miracles', then, were natural cures of hysterical or stress disorders. In the past, to suggest this had been considered tantamount to saying that they were spurious: that the men and women he cured were not really ill. But this is nonsense. Stress disorders are one of nature's expedients to release people from intolerable tensions: it is as if the human mind, finding that evolution has created in disease a useful weapon to control the species, has appropriated it and begun to use it in self-protection. The hysterical patient is ill – just as ill as if a plague had struck him down. But the treatment has to be different: it has to be related to the cause of the disorder – the worries that are creating the disturbance. And Jesus's methods happened to be admirably suited to such cases; never in history, probably, had a therapeutic system been more appropriate to the patients' needs.

Admittedly it is risky to attach too much credence to the gospellers' accounts of Jesus's work as a healer. Much of what they wrote must have been based on hearsay; legends must have attached themselves to Jesus as they do to all successful practitioners. But his technique emerges clearly enough; and it is the same as that which has since been used by generations of healers (for convenience the term 'healer' can be used in its colloquial sense, by contrast with 'doctor'). Its basis was the power of the human imagination: when a person is convinced by suggestion or auto-suggestion that he will be well, he will

The Middle Ages: Christianity

A Byzantine ivory diptych of three of Jesus' healing miracles: the healing of the blind man, the paralytic and the leper

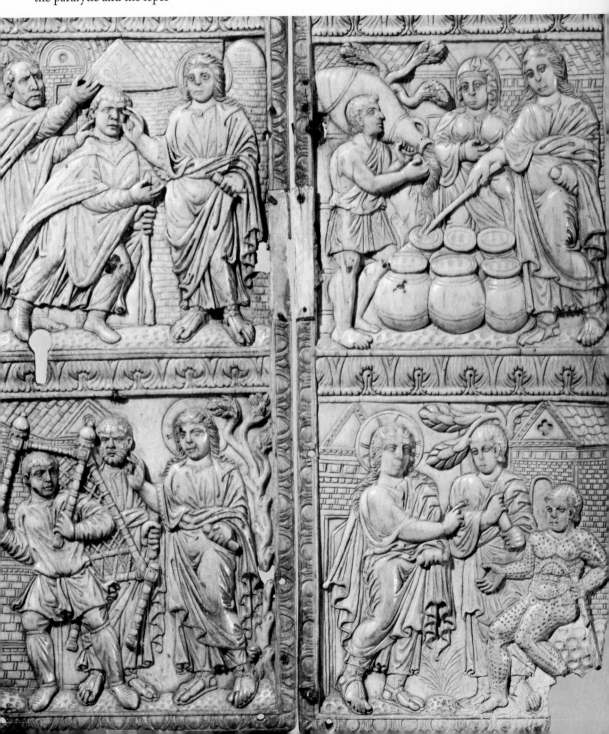

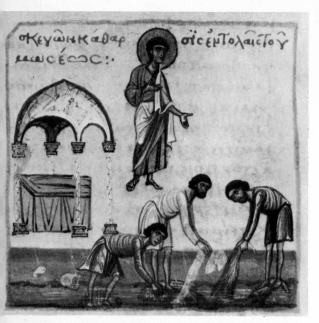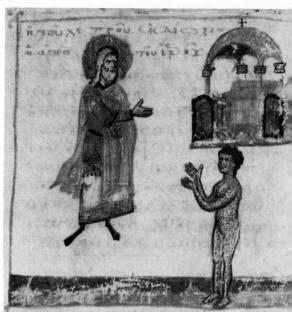

Two miniatures illustrating the Mosaic regulations for preserving health in the Jewish community. *Left:* Soldiers who have sacked a city have to disinfect their clothes before returning into the camp. *Right:* A leper banished from the camp by the priest

Lepers, normally excluded from towns and churches, wait with other sick people outside the church at Eichstadt, where the relics of St Walburga are being transferred, in the hope of a miraculous cure

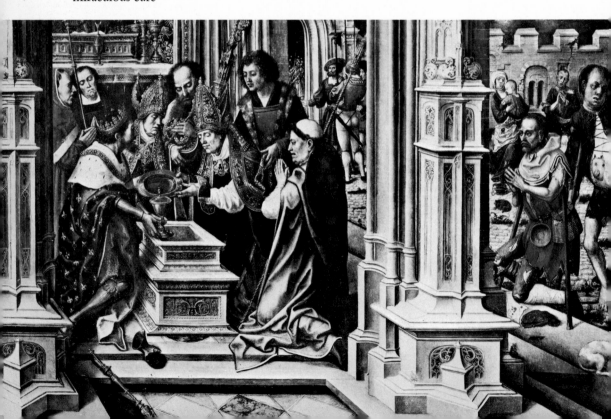

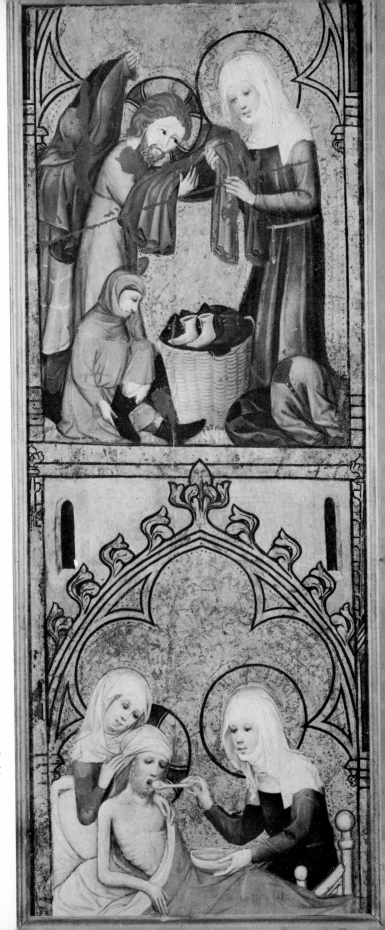

St Elizabeth of Hungary, who
devoted her short life to the service
of the poor, giving alms and feeding
the sick

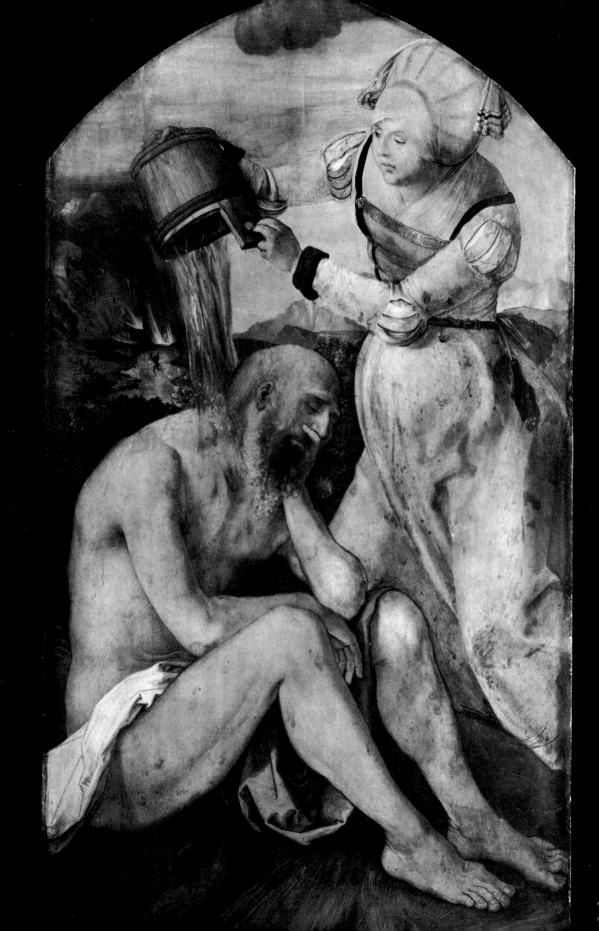

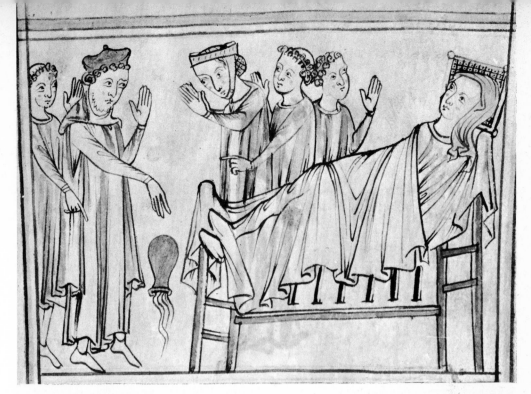

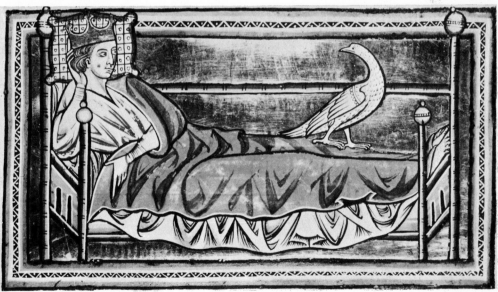

Left: Job and His Wife by Dürer. Christianity considered Job's patient suffering the model attitude to disease

Top: Doctor dropping his urine glass as a sign of unfavourable prognosis. From a medical work by Constantinus Africanus, a monk of Monte Cassino who became one of the leading figures of the Salerno school

Bottom: The Caladrius, from a medieval bestiary, a bird which foretells the course of a patient's illness. As the bird looks towards him, it will draw the sickness out, and the sick king will recover

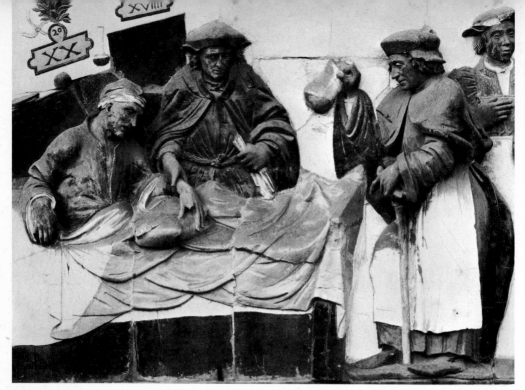

Visiting the Sick from Della Robbia's frieze on the Hospital at Pistoia, illustrating Christian works of mercy. One doctor feels the patient's pulse and the other examines his urine

Part of a plan for the monastery of St Gallen in Switzerland made about 820, showing the infirmary and the doctor's quarters

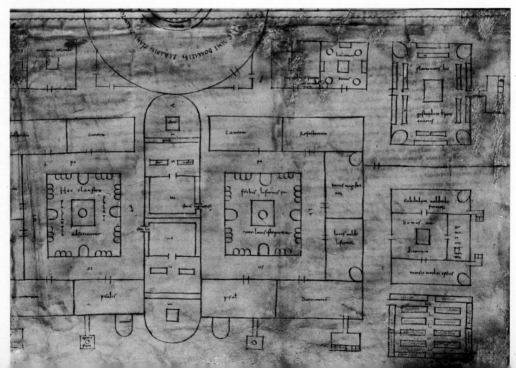

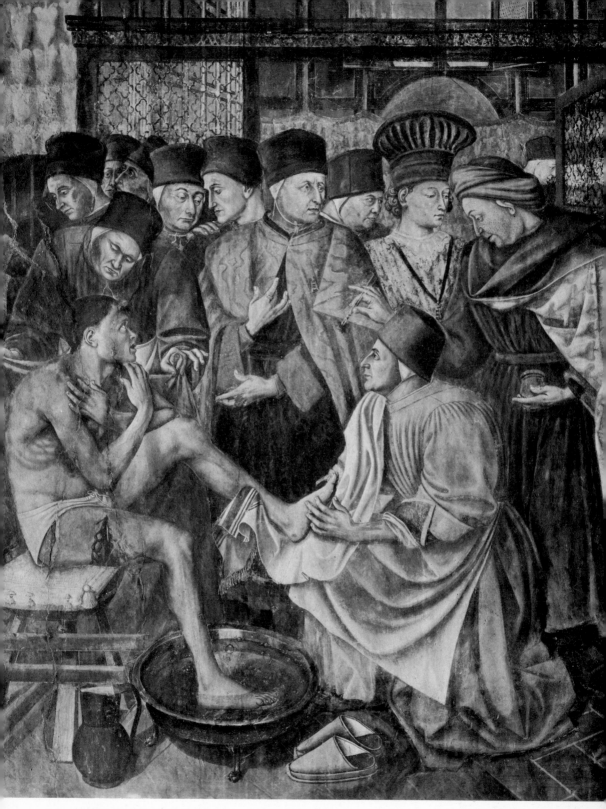

A hospital in the fifteenth century. From a fresco by Domenico di Bartolo in the Hospital of Santa Maria della Scala in Siena

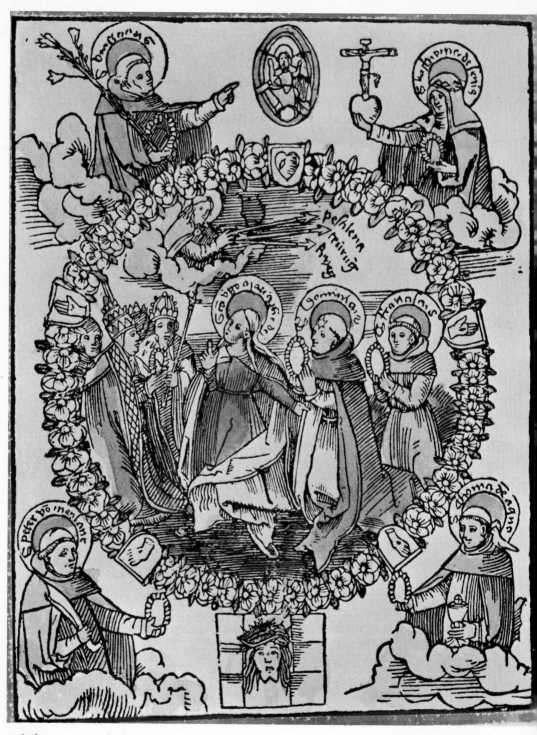

A different aspect of Christianity: this plague sheet shows God afflicting humanity with the triple scourge of pestilence, famine and war, to be mitigated only by intercession through the saints (other things being equal) get well. To touch the imagination, Jesus employed two methods – though he is unlikely to have distinguished between them. One was direct suggestion: 'take up thy bed and walk.' The other was indirect: 'thy sins are forgiven thee.' The force of the indirect method lay in the fact that illness in that community was equated with sinfulness, or lack of faith: the patient's imagination, therefore, had no difficulty in leaping from freedom from sin to freedom from sickness.

It is possible, therefore, to reconcile modern medical theory – now that there is more willingness to accept the need to treat stress disorders as 'real', not just hypochondria, and because of greater awareness of the power of suggestion – with modern Christian theory, which is becoming less wedded to the supernatural element. But another feature of Jesus's healing method remains to be considered; the assumption that there is a specific, though unidentified, healing force, that can be transmitted from one person to others – or, as Jesus believed, from God through him to others, as when the woman touched the hem of his garment; 'Jesus, immediately knowing in himself that virtue had gone out of him, turned about in the press and said "Who touched my clothes?" ' Did he also heal men who were unconscious, or distant, and consequently not amenable to the power of suggestion? Orthodox medicine still refuses to accept the existence of such powers. Yet – as, again, with the Kahunas – it is not now necessary to assume that Jesus must have had supernatural assistance, in order to accept the proposition that suggestion can operate on an *un*conscious level between minds, and therefore at a distance. Recent work on extra-sensory perception has shown that a paranormal broadcasting system, as it were, exists, even if it is not yet clear how it works; and the notion can no longer be dismissed out of hand that some individuals have the power to transmit suggestion – healing or harming – by telepathic means.

Whether Jesus's followers were able adequately to carry on his healing mission may be doubted: but it remained an influential force in Europe until the Renaissance. And in one respect, at least, Christianity left a permanent legacy: an institution which has remained unchanged in some of its conceptions up to the present day: the hospital.

There had been hospitals before: the Aesculapian temples had provided therapeutic centres, and in India Prince Asoka had founded shelters for men and for animals in the third century BC, where medical treatment was available. But for the early Christians – with their need to identify themselves, as Jesus had, with the poor and the sick – hospital work was not so much a charitable gesture as an integral part of the life of the faithful; a way to fulfil the teachings of the Gospels, and to carry on Jesus's healing mission which he himself had handed on to his disciples. 'To do good, and to distribute, forget not': how better could a Christian demonstrate his faith than by helping the poor and the afflicted?

Whether most of the hospitals were really suited to their purpose may be doubted. There were exceptions: the most celebrated of them being St Basil's, Caesarea, opened in 372 as 'a place for the comfort of strangers, both those who are travelling and those who are sick and require treatment' (there were even rehabilitation schemes, so that they could earn a living again after their discharge). But often the convenience of hospitals was more for the donors of charity than for the inmates. It was useful to have a central establishment to which the indigent could be despatched, and where they could be looked after under one roof; it saved the charitably disposed from wasting time and energy looking for them in the slums. And these hospitals often created more problems, and more disease, than they relieved. Unless exceptionally well-managed – and exceptionally well-endowed – they were likely to be squalid, dirty and overcrowded; breeding-grounds for infection.

Work for the sick in those years, therefore, could be dangerous. The women who helped to establish the hospital as an institution were not the Lady Bountifuls of more recent times, sending donations and helping to sell tickets for the annual ball. Fully to identify with Jesus it was necessary for them to put off not merely rank and wealth, but the pride that went with them. If he had washed the feet of beggars, they must realise that no chore could be too laborious or fetid. This required the dedicated spirit of the kind that – according to St Jerome – moved the nobly born Fabiola to work among the patients in the hospital she founded as Astia in 398, out of repentance for her past sins. 'How often did she carry the sick, and wash the pus which others could not bear to look at from their wounds! How often she made their food for them, and sat beside the dying with water to moisten their parched lips!'

Women began to take a more important part in medicine during the Middle Ages than they had been allowed to before. The most imposing was Princess Elizabeth, daughter of the King of Hungary: born early in the thirteenth century; betrothed at the age of four to Ludwig of Thuringia; and married to him ten years later. The pomp of his court repelled her, and she preferred to spend her time among the poor; an activity to which her husband showed himself more tolerant than his courtiers, who were irritated at her contempt for ceremonial and furious to see funds being diverted to charity.

When Ludwig was killed on a crusade they quickly pushed Elizabeth from her estate; and for what remained of her brief life – she died at the age of twenty-four – she devoted herself to good works, and particularly to the sick. Like Fabiola, she won the reputation of having a particular relish for looking after sufferers from the most loathsome diseases. There was something of the religious mania in her, traded on by her notorious confessor Conradin; but at her death, miracles were claimed for her, she was canonised, and her name is perpetuated in many hospitals, as well as in Tannhäuser.

Whether such devotion sprang from mental disorder or from abiding love for fellow human beings – or both – its influence must have been very great. To the poor, accustomed to expect little or nothing when penniless and ill, hospitals must often have appeared God-given, and the men and women who worked in them, saints – as some of them became. The role of the hospital in introducing Christianity to the masses was of decisive importance to the future of the faith. Had the Roman pleb been watching members of an obscure sect, which he knew nothing about, being fed to the lions he would have been left unmoved at their fate. But when some of them had been taken from the hospital where they had been tending his relatives or friends, that was different. This was not lost on the fourth-century Emperor Julian, the Apostate. 'Now we can see', he wrote, 'what it is that makes these Christians such powerful enemies of our gods; it is the brotherly love which they manifest towards strangers, and the sick and the poor'; and he suggested setting up rival hospitals, as a counter-propaganda device.

Such rivals stood little chance. They might have been better equipped and more efficient; but their workers lacked the same dedicated spirit. Probably it was the absence of it that prevented Asoka's from establishing themselves: Buddhism, it has been suggested, failed to put down roots in India, where the seed had first been sown, because Asoka tried to impose it from the top down; whereas Christianity was able to survive and grow in spite of persecution, because of the strength of its roots among the poor.

Hospitals survived the chaos of the collapsing empire: by the sixth century the Church had so far embraced them that they were put on the same basis as monasteries, their privileges and property formally safeguarded. A great many of them must have been makeshift, but descriptions of a few have a modern ring; notably that which was founded and worked in by Margaret of Burgundy in the fifteenth century. A contemporary account describes it as larger than many a cathedral, with massive windows for light and ventilation, cubicles for patients who preferred privacy, tiled floors for simplicity of cleaning, and attractively coloured walls to promote healing.

Many hospitals founded in Europe in the Middle Ages survive: the oldest of them, in Lyons, founded in the sixth century. The first of the still famous London hospitals, St Bartholomew's, was founded early in the twelfth century, St Thomas's following less than a century later. As the Church grew more purse-proud and complacent, the cost of such establishments bore more heavily, and Fabiolas were growing fewer; but by the fifteenth century they had become indispensable, and many of them were taken over by the civic authorities and staffed by lay workers. They were, however, still chiefly places for the sick and indigent to be cared for, rather than treated, in the modern sense of the term. But at least there was somewhere for the sick and indigent to go; and the idea was inculcated that the community owed some responsibility to its less fortunate members.

Plague

Why, then – with Christianity gaining a hold on the people, and with the hospital as an institution becoming perhaps as effective as the church in encouraging conversions – did Christian healing not supplant Galenism? Its power over men's imaginations should have been decidedly stronger, and consequently more effective in the treatment of disease.

One reason for its failure can be traced to the Christian ethic. Christianity had owed a great deal to its success in making the sick, as well as the poor, feel that they were God's children, and his tender care; but at the cost of making disease almost a state of grace. It might indeed be caused by sin; but it also gave the opportunity for redemptions. Through suffering, men and women could learn to share in Jesus's agony on the cross, and to liberate themselves from worldly desires. To be ill, therefore, was an experience to be

cherished; there was even a sense in which to die of an illness was, or a\
could be, better than to survive it. Once it had been firmly established\
life on earth was only a preparation for an eternal reward (provided tha\
was earned) in heaven, the cure of disease became of less importance. I\
patient in hospital recovered suddenly enough for the cure to be accounted\
miraculous, that was useful, because his case could be added to the list of the
appropriate saint who had been invoked, or to whom the hospital had been
dedicated. But 'died after a long illness, bravely borne' might be deemed
even more worthy in the eyes of God. The Recording Angel, watching to see
how the patient comported himself in his decline, might award full marks –
thereby securing the patient a much more rapid passage to heaven than
if he had been out and about, and perhaps sinning, up to the moment of
death.

Christians were also constantly tempted to temporise with orthodox
Galenic medicine – as the Aesculapians had been with their drug-using rivals.
'To buy drugs,' St Bernard of Clairvaux asserted, 'to consult physicians, to
take medicines, befits not religion and is contrary to purity'; theoretically the
faithful observed principles not very different to those of latter-day Christian
Scientists, and based on the advice given in the Epistle of St James, 'Is any sick
among you? Let him call for the elders of the Church, and let them pray over
him, anointing him with oil in the name of the Lord; and the prayer of faiths
shall save the sick, and the Lord shall raise him up.' But the use of herbs was
permitted for everyday disorder; they were grown for this purpose in monastery gardens; and monks often found themselves, without intending to,
acting as general practitioners for the neighbourhood, prescribing simple
drugs and even performing minor surgery. This could be justified because it
helped to keep the monastery solvent and popular locally, in much the same
way as the distillation of liqueurs was later to do; but it eroded faith in God's
therapeutic activities.

By the twelfth century, Christian medicine had so far slipped from the pre-
cepts of its founder that the Council of Rheims was compelled to admit that
an 'evil and detestable custom' had established itself: 'monks and regular
clergy, despising the rules of the blessed Benedict and Augustine, practise law
and medicine for worldly profit.' Medicine was regarded as being even more
deplorable than law; offenders, it was decided, would be excommunicated.
But that the threat failed to have an effect is clear from the fact that it had

constantly to be repeated, with particular injunctions against the practice by clerics and monks of surgery. It was too late: the Church had in effect come to terms with Galenism – even finding its authoritarianism distinctly congenial.

That clerics were practising as physicians and surgeons is revealing; by the end of the Middle Ages, evidently, confidence in Christian healing must have been lost. And it is easy to understand why. Jesus's methods might work in the tightly knit, devout Hebrew community of his time, where the scrupulous observance of regulations about public and private hygiene reduced the rate of infectious diseases – against which his methods could not have been very effective – but increased the rate of stress disorders – against which they were, or at least, could be, effective. But in the Middle Ages not only did Christianity lose its early unity – splitting up as it did into warring sects, each denouncing the other as wicked and heretical, thereby loosening its hold on the imaginations of the faithful; it also had to contend with a different pattern of disease.

The most serious threat by this time were not stress disorders, but epidemics – malaria, typhus, bubonic plague, and others unidentified. Suggestion does not entirely lack a therapeutic potential in epidemics: recent research has suggested that in some, notably in cholera, it may play a significant part. But it usually worked *against* survival, because fear operated more effectively on the imagination than hope. Amulets containing wolf dung might have armed people against less lethal disorders; against the dreaded plague they were useless. It may well be true, as has so often been suggested, that in some epidemics, fear was the executioner-in-chief.

Epidemics had been known before, but they had been surprisingly infrequent, even among armies. In the declining years of the Roman Empire, they began to increase, culminating in the great plague of Justinian in 541, so vividly described by Procopius. The first symptom was slight fever, followed by glandular swellings under the armpits and elsewhere in the body. Some patients went into a delirium, others into a coma; the most unlucky of all were those who retained possession of their faculties, and died in agony:

Some died at once; others after many days; and the bodies of some broke out with black blisters the size of a lentil. These did not live after one day, but died at once; and many were quickly killed by the vomiting of blood which attacked them. Physicians could not tell which cases were light and which severe, and no remedies availed.

Though admitting that accurate estimate was impossible, Gibbon conjectured that for over a period of three months there must have been between five and ten thousand deaths a day at Constantinople alone: whole cities had to be abandoned. 'The triple scourge of war, pestilence and famine afflicted the subjects of Justinian; and his reign is disgraced by a visible decrease of the human species which has never been regained in some of the fairest countries of the globe.'

At the time, it was commonly assumed that the signal had been given by God: epidemics reflected his wrath – his punishment for mankind and its perverse wickedness. And there is a sense, Zinsser suggested, in which this interpretation was not far off the mark. In its decline, and particularly during Justinian's attempt to restore it from Byzantium, the Empire was, for various reasons, inherently epidemic-prone. Justinian was trying to impose his rule on unwilling peoples by force of arms; but authority at the centre was corrupt, and the poison eventually corrupted the whole. Incessant warfare at the frontier, political oppression within its boundaries, and civil disaffection in and around the seat of government, all led to the kind of inefficiently run, disorganised and dissatisfied society of a kind which is custom-made to encourage the spread of an infectious disease, when one is introduced.

With the discovery of microbes, the notion of plagues being a kind of judgment on a community or a continent has gone out of fashion. It seems an altogether more rational explanation that Europeans fell easy victims for much the same reasons that Red Indians were later killed off by viruses introduced from Europe, or that rabbits were slaughtered by artificially induced myxomatosis. In other parts of the world, the plague had been endemic, so communities had built up resistance to it; but when it reached Europe, the virus found people with no immunity, and it was much more destructive.

But this does not provide the whole answer. 'We know the bacillus that causes plague,' Sigerist argued, 'we know how it is transmitted from rodents to man, and how an epidemic spreads along the highways of traffic. Yet we do not know why Europe was devastated by two pandemics of plague in the sixth and fourteenth centuries, but experienced no serious outbreak of the disease during the intervening eight hundred years, although Europe had very close and intimate contacts with the Orient during the crusades.' And recently studies of epidemiology have been coming round to the conclusion that though viruses may be the agents of an epidemic, they are not its sole cause: ordinarily, there must be some predisposition in the individual or the community.

Whether the predisposition is constitutional or environmental (or both) remains uncertain; nor has anybody provided a satisfying reason why plagues should have struck as inconsequentially as they did, or why some should have been so much more destructive than others. What made the people of Europe, for example, so susceptible to the bubonic plague when it appeared in the form of the Black Death? It swept in from Asia and Africa in 1348; as Boccaccio described it:

... in men and women alike there appeared at the beginning of the malady certain swellings, either on the groin or under the armpits, some of the size of an apple; others more like an egg, and these the vulgar named 'plague-boils'. From these two parts the plague boils quickly proceeded to appear indifferently in every part of the body. After a while, the fashion of the contagion began to change, into black or livid blotches which appeared in many first on the arms and then on every other part of the person; in some large and sparse, in others small and thick sown. But just as the plague boils had been from the first (and still were) a certain indication of coming death, so were these blotches to everyone they afflicted.

A quarter of the entire population of Europe, it was conservatively estimated, was wiped out by the Black Death; and though no later outbreak of the plague reached the same serious proportions, frequent outbreaks followed.

So though the Black Death's destructiveness may have been due to a lethal species of virus encountering people who had not acquired immunity, and running through them much as smallpox and measles were later to do when exported to the New World, the later outbreaks, and epidemics of other kinds, are probably more easily accountable for by the general condition of society – psychological and moral, as well as economic and social. There are innumerable indications that mental as well as physical derangements were highly contagious – using that term in its colloquial sense.

The earliest intimations of the plague of Justinian, according to Procopius, were a kind of haunting by phantoms, who threatened death to individuals, in dreams or in waking visions; and death would follow. In the later Middle Ages, outbreaks of St Vitus's Dance, or tarantism – the dancing mania – became common. The most reasonable hypothesis to account for them is that they were, in Zinsser's words, 'mass hysterias, brought on by terror and

Opposite: Miraculous Cure by a Saintly Bishop.
Tyrolean school, *c.* 1500

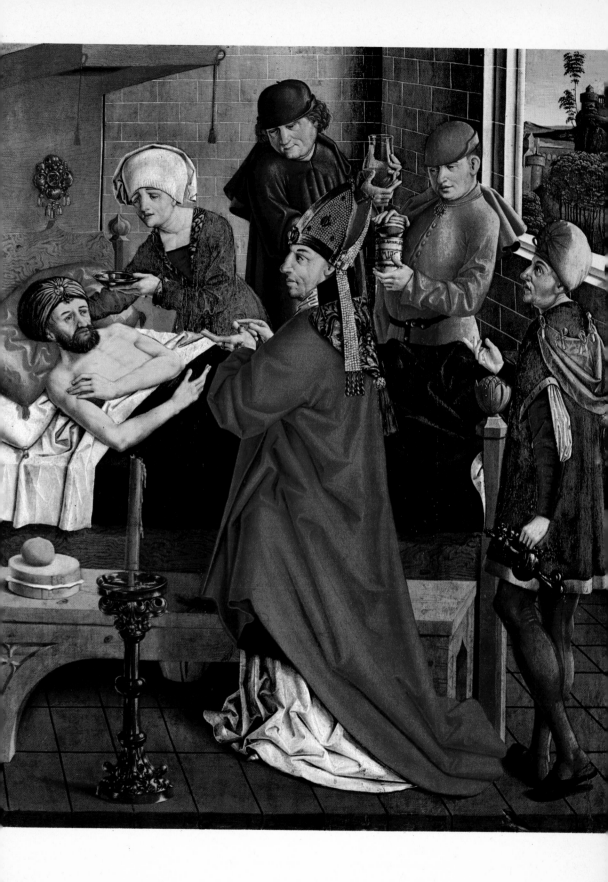

despair, in populations oppressed, famished and wretched to a degree almost unimaginable today'. It was as if nature had decided that the human race was showing itself to be one of her evolutionary failures; and, having exhausted her available supply of physical diseases to wipe out her mistake, she had recalled her expedient to control the lemming population, and adapted it against humanity. References to groups of people being afflicted by the dancing mania are not uncommon in the earlier Middle Ages; but the best documented of the epidemics began at Aix la Chapelle in 1374, and was given the name of St John's, or St Vitus's, dance. In his *Epidemics of the Middle Ages*, the German authority, Professor J. F. Hecker, described how the victims

formed circles hand in hand, appearing to have lost all control over their senses; and continued dancing, regardless of the bystanders, for hours together in wild delirium, until at length they fell to the ground in a state of exhaustion. They then complained of extreme oppression, and groaned as if in the agonies of death . . . while dancing they neither saw nor heard, being insensible to external impressions through the senses, but were haunted by visions, their fancies conjuring up spirits whose names they shrieked out; and for some of them afterwards where the disease was completely developed, the attack commenced with epileptic convulsions. Those affected fell to the ground senseless, panting and labouring for breath. They foamed at the mouth; then, suddenly springing up, began their dance amidst strange contortions.

The dancing mania was a kind of communal fit; the most striking example in history of epidemic hysteria. 'Whom the gods wish to destroy, they first make mad'; probably some of the crusades, notably Peter the Hermit's and the Children's Crusade, were really disguised versions of the same affliction. Hecker believed that the epidemics were brought on as a result both of the physical effects of the great plagues, and of the moral degradation that accompanied them. 'Security of property there was none; arbitrary will everywhere prevailed; corruption of morals and rude power rarely met with even a feeble opposition . . . if we take into consideration that among the numerous bands, many wandered about whose consciences were tormented with the recollection of the crimes which they had committed during the prevalence of the Black Death, we shall comprehend how their despair sought relief in the intoxication of an artificial delirium.' Koestler, too, has since suggested that the Middle Ages were particularly conducive to this mass

hysteria because of the chronic and insoluble mental conflict which confronted people unable to resolve the contradiction between their faith in a
Christian code, and the hideous reality of the world they lived in. Surely – their
feeling must often have been – no merciful God, on Jesus's model, could have
been so callous as to allow his children to suffer so.

The victims of the dancing mania were treated either by swaddling them,
like babies – a primitive version of the straitjacket which was not really
treatment, but designed simply to prevent them from being a danger to
themselves and others; or exorcism, which was rarely effective, and difficult
to carry out in the face of a maniacal mob. The only recorded successfu
form of treatment came from Italy, where the mania was known as tarantism, because it was attributed to the bite of the tarantula spider. The belief
arose there that cure could be effected by homeopathic means; with the help
of a hectic dance to vigorous music (the tarantella), victims of the 'bite' – or
the mania – were often able to throw off its effects. Interestingly, this was
the same belief that the followers of Pythagoras had brought to Italy over
a thousand years before; perhaps it had lingered on there in folk lore. Some
commentators have doubted whether the method was effective, but it may
well have performed the same kind of function as electric-shock treatment.
Sufferers, given what amounted to an artificially induced fit, were relieved
of the torments of the real one.

Ordinarily, though, there was no attempt at treatment. 'Neither the
advice of any physician,' Boccaccio wrote, 'nor the virtue of any medicine
prevailed.' The plague, he and his contemporaries assumed, must be the
consequence either of an unfortunate conjunction of heavenly bodies, or 'of
our own iniquitous dealings, being sent down upon mankind for our correction by the just wrath of God'; and if God were responsible, there was not
much point in any evasive action, except penitence and prayer. But the
heavenly bodies might be circumvented by magic; so the ranks of orthodoxy
were supplemented by great numbers of men and women practising variations of sorcery. No doubt many of them were quacks in the derogatory
sense of the term; but to work among the plague-stricken, or even in communities not yet attacked but at risk, must have been hazardous, however
lucrative; probably many of the sorcerers really believed in their methods.
Sometimes, these methods may have been as effective as any that Christians
were using; but by this time sorcery had little more power than Christianity

to stimulate the public imagination. By the end of the Middle Ages Galenism was establishing itself as orthodoxy, accepted by Church and State, and practised by trained physicians.

Galen Restored

For the Christian to consult a lay physician might indicate uncertainty about his priest's powers; but the division of labour had not been entirely illogical, as the lay physician worked on a lower level. Ordinarily he occupied a status roughly equivalent to the present-day masseur or physiotherapist; he was a medical auxiliary. Although the range of services required from him could be much wider than for present-day auxiliaries, he was often untrained – except through a form of apprenticeship, assisting his predecessor. He was also often illiterate, his knowledge based largely on folk lore about herbs and their appropriate incantations.

Organised lay medicine in Europe, however, began to emerge with the School of Salerno, which established itself in the eleventh century. It cannot be claimed as the first medical school: Alexandria, in the time of Hierophilus and Erasistratus was an earlier and in some ways more impressive example. But from Alexandria no written records remain; we know of what was accomplished there only from hearsay and legend. The information about the Salerno school is less scanty.

Salerno had been popular as a health resort in Roman times; and it seems possible that it owed its medical school to a revival of this reputation, coupled with the fact that in the nearby monastery, Monte Cassino, there was a collection of old medical works which had been preserved there, and which provided the Salerno school with its texts. The school also produced some texts of its own, of which a couple have retained their interest: one, indeed – the *Regimen Sanitatis Salernitanum* – has often been described as the most popular medical textbook ever written. Its date and authorship remain uncertain; but its Hippocratic charm remains:

> Use three doctors still, First Dr Quiet
> Next, Dr Merry-man and Dr Diet.

The basis was humoral:

> Four Humors reign within our body wholly
> And these compared to four elements
> The Sanguine, Choler, Phlegm and Melancholy.

The other famous Salerno work – credited to Trotula, the 'Dame Trot' of fairly tale – dealt with gynaecology and other matters of interest to women. This was of some importance, as in the early Middle Ages women could only be attended when in labour by women; and the advice available for them had been limited largely to a survey of the relative efficacy of rival charms or incantations. *De passionibus mulierum* was needed, therefore, not merely for midwives, but also for doctors, now that the prejudice was subsiding. The instructions follow the familiar pattern: scraps of sound commonsense mingled with lore, prejudice and magic. Doubts have been expressed that the author was really a woman, but the treatise has a distinctly feminine bias. A lip salve was prescribed for girls whose lips have been cracked by the too hungry kisses of her lover: as for the lover, if insufficiently virile, asses' excrement was recommended.

These Salerno texts preserved a remarkable popularity; they were reprinted so frequently up to the end of the sixteenth century that they must have been in household use, and not just literary curiosities. They reflected, and must to some extent have encouraged, the trend away from both religion and magic in everyday medicines. Disease was attributed to natural causes, not to divine displeasure; the saints were not invoked; and astrology and incantations absent. For all their limitations, these Salerno texts can reasonably be regarded as early intimations of the scientific revolution that used to be regarded as dating from the Renaissance.

The Salerno school can also claim to have attracted the interest of the most remarkable figure of his era: Frederick II of Hohenstaufen – 'Stupor Mundi', the prototype of the Renaissance man. His father had captured and sacked Salerno in 1194, but the school survived, and during his reign Frederick issued instructions about the award of degrees there. He was interested in medicine – as in much else; savants and practitioners flocked to his court as they had once to Chosroes', including Michael Scot, who introduced Europe to Aristotle's biology. Although Frederick was himself rationalist by inclination, rationalism in that age was anti-clerical rather than anti-mystic: the fact that Scot was chiefly interested in the arcane, a sorcerer rather than a physician, was no bar to Frederick's patronage.

Among Frederick's correspondents was Peter of Spain – so called, though he was of Portuguese origin; the author of some medical treatises, and the only doctor to become Pope. He owed his elevation to the Papacy to the death in rapid succession of three predecessors; as physician to the Vatican he might have been regarded with some suspicion, but legend has it that the cardinals were anxious to appoint somebody with a prospect of a longer tenure of office, and they felt his clinical knowledge might be better exercised upon himself – especially as a prophecy had promised him long life. It proved incorrect; the roof of a palace he was constructing for himself fell in on him a few months later, to the undisguised relief of the orthodox, who regarded him as anti-Christ.

Although Frederick favoured men of esoteric views in his court, his attitude to public health appears to have been eminently practical. In the twelfth century his grandfather, Roger II of Sicily, had already deemed it necessary to regulate the practice of the new, lay medicine; Frederick amplified Roger's regulations, insisting that anybody who wished to practise as a doctor (the term began to be used at this time to designate a member of the medical profession) must first pass an examination, so that 'the king's subjects should not incur danger through the inexperience of their physicians'. Frederick's rules have a modern ring: a five years' training course was specified, and medical students also had to undertake a year's apprenticeship. It was also laid down that the doctor must not be a partner with an apothecary, in case this should tempt him to prescribe too many or too expensive drugs; the selling price and the quality of drugs was also controlled, with inspectors to check that they had been made according to the prescription, and offered for sale only in that condition.

Again, the existence of such regulations is not necessarily an indication that the discipline they seek to enforce will be observed; but Frederick's have a confident air about them, as if they really were designed to protect the public from unscrupulous exploitation – rather than simply to give the public that impression, while doing nothing effective. Certainly this would accord with the general picture of enlightened Hohenstaufen competence. And although after Frederick's death his empire disintegrated, the pattern he established was remembered and copied elsewhere; as when a century later Henry V laid down similar regulations for England, insisting that anybody who practised physic must present himself at a university for examination, and obtain a degree – or risk punishment by the Privy Council. When the medical profession eventually began to establish itself in its present form, in the nineteenth century, it was basically Frederick's principles that were accepted and enacted.

Yet his ideas of how to regulate the practice of medicine, though admirably intentioned, were to have some unfortunate results. If an aspiring doctor had to undertake a five years' training course, he had to be taught something during that time; and the easiest way for his professors to teach him was to prescribe certain books and examine him on his knowledge of them. Orthodoxy prescribed Galen, the key to the examination door for nearly four centuries; and though other authorities forced their way in, notably Avicenna, what the medical student could learn from them was limited. He might if he were energetic become as well versed as Chaucer's physician in the works of Hippocrates, Galen and Avicenna – and in the intricacies of the humoral theory, in astrology, and in sorcery. But this did not make him a good doctor, and Chaucer, although he admired his doctor, clearly did not like him:

> Gold stimulates the heart, or so we're told
> He therefore had a special love of gold

With universities and medical schools beginning to spring up all over Europe, medical teaching became more formalised. Even if the textbooks had been far better for purposes of instruction than they were, the academic trend would still have been stultifying; but as Galen and Avicenna had provided not so much textbooks as encyclopedias of, for the most part, contentious, incorrect and muddled information, warped into a fallacious theory, the effect was numbing.

By the Middle Ages, academic interest had shifted from the humors themselves to what were assumed to be their psychological counterparts; patients were classified according to temperament, sanguine, phlegmatic, melancholy or choleric. This represented an advance, for it was at least possible to estimate a man's temperament; whereas there had been no way, other than guesswork or divination, of diagnosing the state of his bodily humors. But it did not necessarily provide any more satisfactory a basis for deciding on treatment: the decision how to try to cure an illness still had to be taken on arbitrary grounds – and treatments could be arbitrary indeed.

Galen had tended to favour polypharmacy: so did his successors. The more ingredients that went into a prescription the more effective it was thought likely to be; so the prescriber of involved doses was admired – not least by the apothecaries. And for lack of a more subtle diagnostic system the drugs were usually administered on the principle of contraries. This at least had the merit that the patient got the impression something was being done for him: if he had a fever, a drug was prescribed to lower his temperature – which seemed sensible: if he felt relaxed, a constricting drug would be prescribed, and vice versa, on the Methodics' principle – which seemed logical. When it was not clear what was the matter with him, bleeding became the standard treatment; the assumption being that he must be suffering from a plethora, and that bleeding would relieve it ('cupping' – drawing up a section of the skin by an artificial vacuum into a small cup – was also frequently prescribed, on the same principle).

Because they gave the illusion of having a rational basis, these methods may have worked well enough, through suggestion, for some disorders. But they had the disadvantage that they were too simple: patients were not always sufficiently impressed. So, as time went on, they came to be embellished with ritual. The bleeding (or cupping) had to be done in a certain way, at a certain time, in a certain part of the body, according to the patient's horoscope or the season of the year.

Medicine, then, remained firmly stuck in its antiquated groove. Occasionally somebody arose who questioned the authorities' infallibility; in England in the thirteenth century Roger Bacon pleaded for a new approach, based on original research rather than on acceptance of traditional authority; and as he had some remarkable hunches about the future – the most celebrated being his forecast of the machine age and of X-rays – he might have had much to contribute if he had been allowed to follow his own prescription. But a questioning attitude was not welcomed by his superiors in the Church, who gave Bacon plenty of time to meditate on his ideas in prison – a punishment that was also given at the end of the century to Peter of Abano, for his attempts to bring together religion, philosophy and medicine in a new rational synthesis. Peter suggested that the healing miracles of Jesus might not be miraculous – that Lazarus might have been raised not from the dead, but from a trance. His views were condemned as blasphemous; but he died while on trial before the Inquisition, so that although they pronounced him guilty and pronounced the inevitable sentence, it was his corpse that burned at the stake.

7

THE RENAISSANCE

Paracelsus

THE crucial date for the birth of the Renaissance, it has been suggested, is 1443, when a manuscript was found in a Milan church which turned out to be part of Celsus's encyclopedia, lost since Roman times. Most of it has still never been found; but the part discovered happened to be *De re medicina*, written during the reign of the emperor Tiberius, and presenting an absorbing picture of the medical theory and practice of his time. Like the Hippocratic writings, to which it bore some resemblance, *De re medicina* was probably a compilation, comprising earlier material from Greece and elsewhere; but, both because it was the earliest medical work known other than the Hippocratic writings, and because of the beauty of its Latin prose, which entranced scholars, its impact was considerable. And among those who were to be attracted by its Hippocratic purity, a contrast to the elaborate structures of Galen and Avicenna, was Theophrastus Bombast von Hohenheim, born near Zurich in 1493 – the year after Columbus's discovery of America.

Styling himself Paracelsus, von Hohenheim was to become – in Osler's phrase – the Luther of medicine: 'the very incarnation of revolt. At a period when authority was paramount, and men blindly followed old leaders, when to stray from the beaten track in any field of knowledge was a damnable heresy, he stood out boldly for independent study and the right of private judgment.' Boldly is not quite the appropriate word: Paracelsus was not so much a man of decision as – in Browning's description – 'a man possessed by a fire' – by a demon.

The son of a doctor, Paracelsus decided to adopt the same career; at some point in his studies he realised that orthodox medicine was not so much wrong as irrelevant and meaningless: 'when I saw that nothing resulted from

Plagues and Epidemics

Three doctors at the bedside of a plague victim, who points to the plague-boil under his armpit

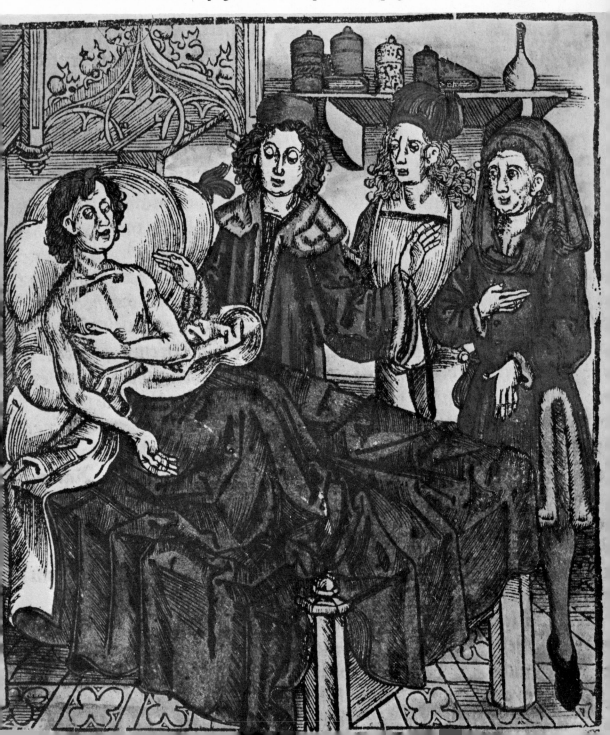

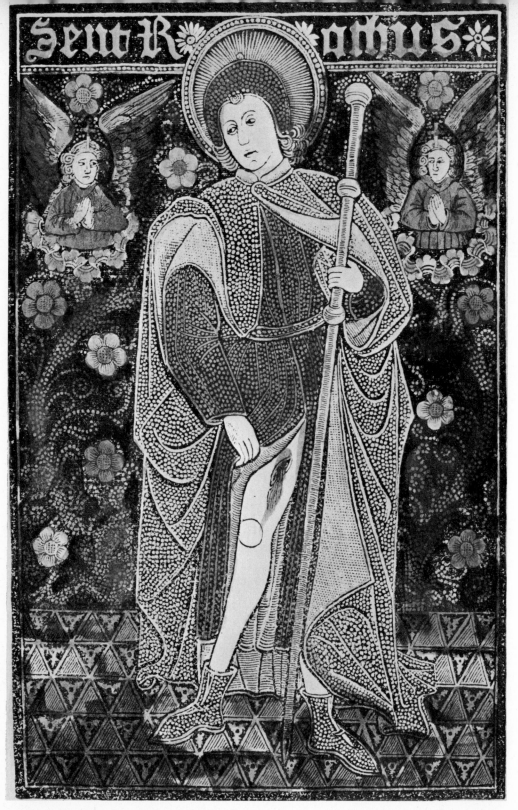

St Roch, shown on this plague-sheet from the Rhineland, was born at Montpellier and studied medicine there. He caught the plague in Italy when he went there to give help to the sick during the Black Death

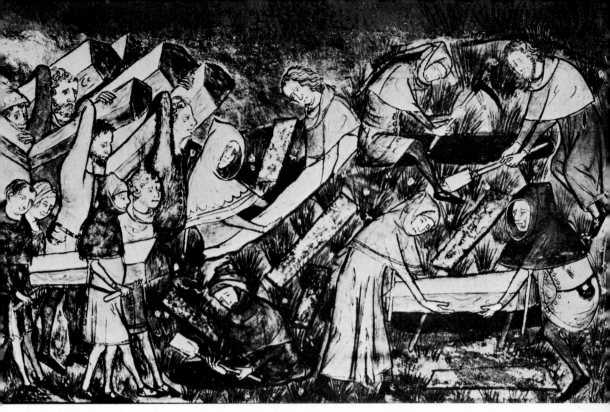

Miniature showing the burial of victims of the Black Death at Tournai in 1349

Animals and humans dead or dying of the plague, an illustration (*c.* 1520) by Hans Weiditz to Petrarch's *De Remediis*

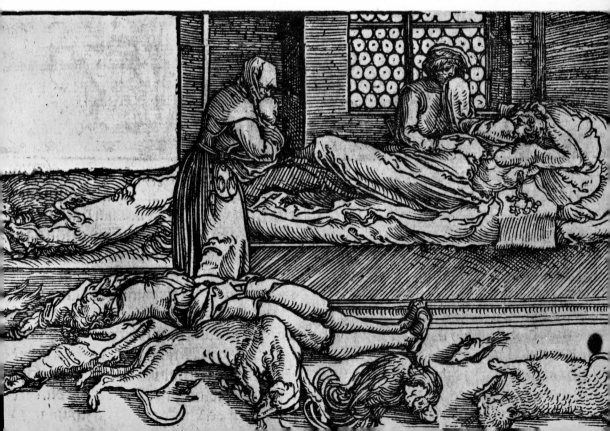

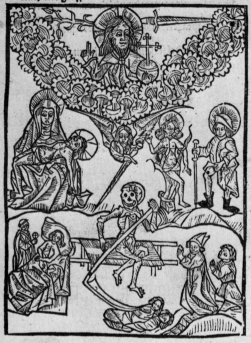

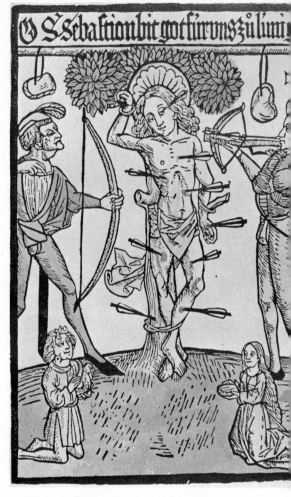

Left: Title-page of Philip Culmacher's *Regimen* (*c.* 1495), one of the earliest printed treatises suggesting ways of preventing the plague

Right: St Sebastian, as well as St Roch, was invoked by plague sufferers: a man and woman bring their offerings of food to the pilgrimage shrine of Linange in Lorraine

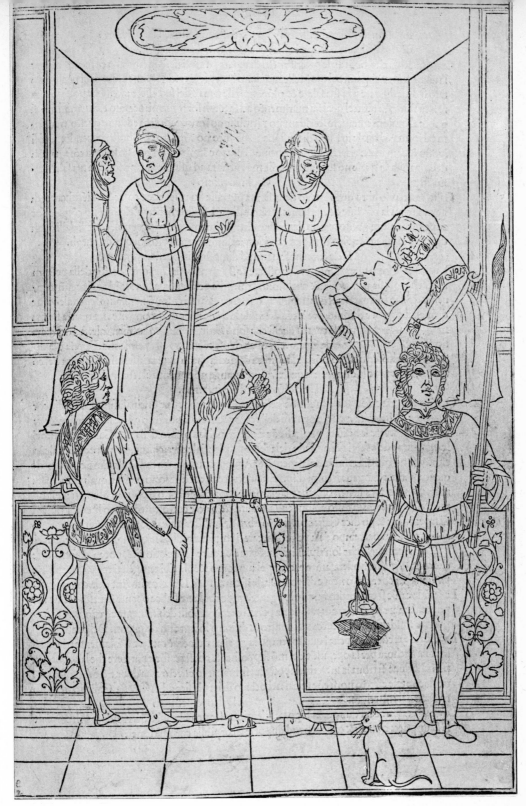

A doctor, feeling the pulse of a plague patient, protects himself by holding an impregnated sponge to his nose, while his servants burn aromatics

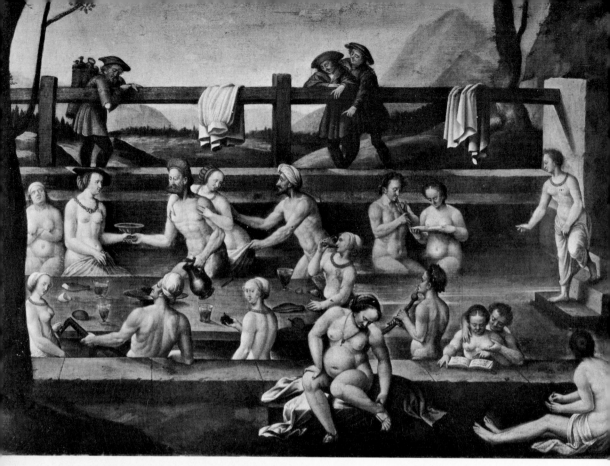

The later Middle Ages were afflicted with a mania for bathing. The origins may have been hygienic, but communal baths such as this in the thermal springs at Leukerbad only increased the spread of contagious diseases, and particularly syphilis

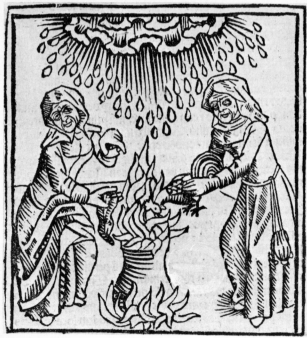

Left: Witches working a spell. From Molitor's *De Lamiis*, published shortly after the *Malleus Maleficarum*

Right: Hans Baldung Grien's painting of *Two Witches* (1523) illustrates the erotic element in witchcraft in popular imagination

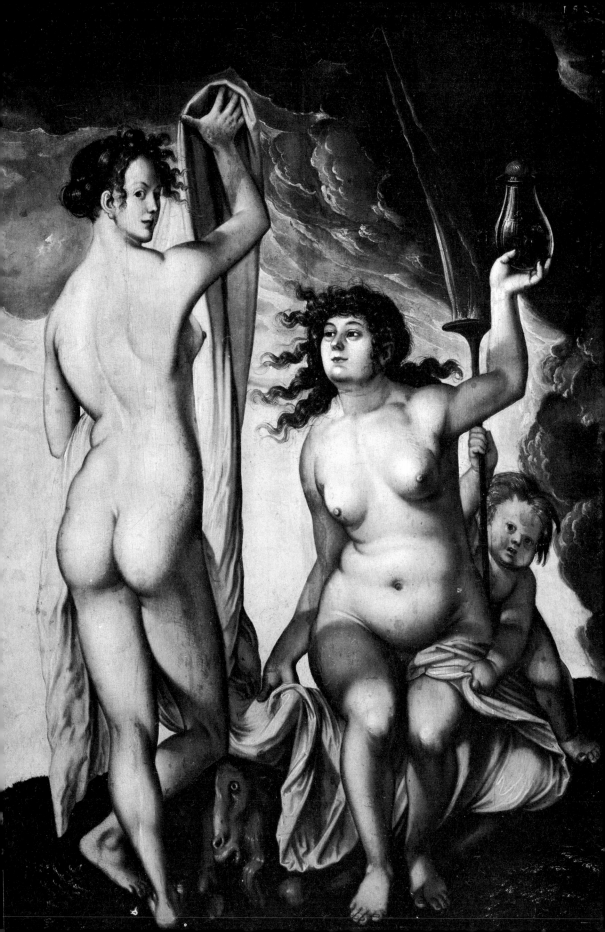

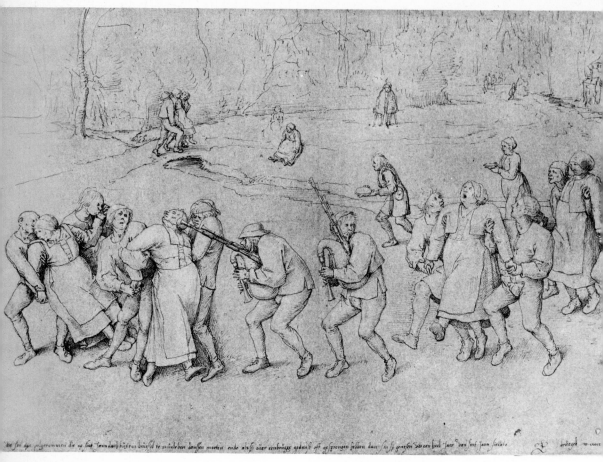

Drawing by Brueghel (1564)
showing women suffering from the
dancing mania, restrained by their
companions, on a pilgrimage to
Meulebeke in western Flanders

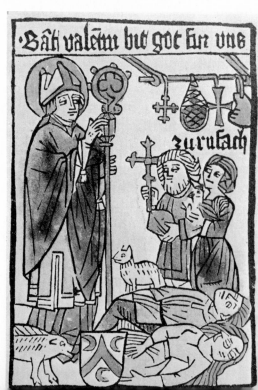

The patron saint of epileptics was
Valentine of Rufach, here invoked
by pilgrims bringing offerings of
food

their practice but killing and laming, that they deemed most complaints incurable, and that they administered scarcely anything but syrup laxatives,
purgatives and oatmeal gruel, with everlasting clysters, I determined to
abandon such a miserable art and seek truth elsewhere.' He began on his
travels, all over Europe and the Middle East, questioning, arguing, experimenting. When he returned to Europe, ten years later, and settled down to
practise in Strasbourg, these travels gave him not only experience but a
mystique; he quickly established a reputation which reached the celebrated
printer Frobenius in Basle, suffering from agonising pains in his right leg following an accident some years before. The doctors wished to amputate; but
Frobenius first called in Paracelsus, who was able to cure him without recourse to the knife. He also successfully treated Frobenius's still more famous
guest, Erasmus; and when the Basle authorities, impressed, offered him the
post of town physician, Paracelsus had the opportunity to embark on a
profitable conventional career.

One of the duties, however, attached to the post was lecturing to the local
medical students; and Paracelsus could not resist the temptation to expound
his heretical opinions. He brought along the works of Galen and Avicenna
only to burn them; and he took care to deliver his denunciation of them in
the vernacular, instead of in the conventional Latin, which to the local
doctors made his heresy seem the more heinous. So far from supporting him,
his students were alarmed at his unconventionality, which might jeopardise
their careers: and when the town council proved as parsimonious as Hamelin's
had been to its pied piper, Paracelsus left Basle in bitterness, to resume his
wanderings. His egotism and bluntness made it difficult for him to find any-
where to settle down: the classic phrase with which he contemptuously dismissed the doctors of his day, 'they have gone, and still go, around the art of
medicine like a cat around hot porridge', did not endear him to his colleagues.
And though he found time to write a great deal before his death in 1541, it
was but rarely that he could persuade anybody to publish it.

As a result, much of his work was not published till some years after his
death; and this has presented the usual tedious difficulties about deciding
what to count as his, and what to attribute to the revisions and interpolations
of over-zealous disciples, anxious to give their own ideas his sanction – or
antagonists, seeking to discredit him by putting in his mouth ideas they
detested. Still, a reasonably clear picture of his thought has emerged.

Medicine, Paracelsus believed, rested on four pillars. First, astronomy: man was the microcosm, the universe was the macrocosm, and fully to understand man it is necessary to understand the workings of the cosmos. Second, natural science – including geography (his travels had made him a believer in the importance of regional variations in disease). Third, chemistry – the refinement and application of natural substances for purposes of treatment. Fourth, love: only a virtuous, unselfish man, he asserted, could hope to be a good physician.

Substitute 'God' for the cosmos, and Paracelsus's four-pillared structure could have passed for orthodoxy; but it was not a system of medicine, only a blueprint for one. The test for any medical systematiser is how he relates his theoretical structure to the needs of patients. To Paracelsus, Galenism was useless because it failed to do so: and he proceeded to construct one of his own – at first sight not very promising, as it was based on the assumption that there were three elements, mercury, sulphur, and salt. But the theoretical foundation was less important than what Paracelsus proceeded to construct on it. The life force, he insisted, was all important: the 'archeus' he called it, a 'radiating essence' which through the imagination, could produce healthy or unhealthy effects. Imagination, that was the important thing: 'the character of the physician acts more powerfully upon the patient than all the drugs administered' because it was his character which touched the patient's imagination. In the same way, a sick imagination could cause disease: 'conscience overcomes the guilty one; envy and hatred have similar effects: thereby many sicknesses of many different kinds can be brought on. Therefore you should apply treatment not as in ordinary diseases; you should treat the psyche, for it is the psyche that here lies sick.'

With his hypnotic personality, Paracelsus might have established himself just as Galen had, acquiring fame and fortune. But here, his demon stepped in, refusing to allow him to embrace his self-interest. When Paracelsus had a hunch, he had to follow it, and to express it, whether or not it fitted with his system – and his prospects. He was constantly experimenting with drugs, for example, and introducing new ones, particularly minerals – laudanum, the opium derivative, was his idea; and Wootton, the chronicler of pharmacy – not given to such eulogy – described him as 'perhaps the greatest emancipator of the human race from the chains of slavish obedience to authority in the past thousand years'. But unlike Galen, Paracelsus refused to be impressed by his contributions to the *materia medica*. He did not approve of the use of drugs, except in emergencies; and when he used them he preferred simplicity. Polypharmacy was abhorrent to him – as were those who traded on it: 'apothecaries are my enemies because I will not empty their boxes. My recipes are simple and do not call for forty or fifty ingredients. I seek not to enrich the apothecaries, but to cure the sick.'

To cure the sick, he realised – like the Hippocrat he was – the essential need was to sustain the life force. 'In nature's battle against disease the physician is but the helper, who furnishes nature with weapons: nature is the physician.' He kept his eyes open for the subtle ways in which the life force might be being impeded, without people realising it. His early experience among miners had made him aware of the hazards of occupational diseases, which he was the first to elucidate; and his travels had given him an appreciation of the influence of geography and environment on the disease pattern – as well as the powers of observation which led him to make such a discovery as the link between cretinism and goitre.

Unlike Hippocrates, Paracelsus was not content simply to seek for ways to enable the life force to operate more freely. There must, he felt, be some way to stimulate it; and the best way, he came to the conclusion, was through love. He was himself a truculent, cross-grained man without, so far as can be judged, much charity in his character; but he realised objectively that here was a potent therapeutic force, operating through faith, and 'capable of making for itself every herb – an invisible nettle, an invisible celandine, an invisible trioll; everything that grows in terrestial nature, the power of belief can likewise bring' – with its counterpart: 'the power of belief can likewise create every sickness.'

Almost every branch of medicine has since been forced to recognise its debt to Paracelsus: but the greatest beneficiary is psychiatry. 'The present day clergy in Europe', he wrote, 'attribute mental diseases to ghostly beings and spirits; we are not inclined to believe them'; and he went on to explain that diseases which deprive men of their reason originated, in his experience, out of some fault in their inner personalities – though he was careful to differentiate between mania which arose from this internal cause, and that which emerged as a side-effect of some other illness. His differentiation between the imbecile and the psychopath was equally in advance of his time; 'a trailblazer in empirical psychology and psychotherapy,'

75

Jung was to describe him; 'in his own way he took the phenomena of the soul into consideration, as none of the great physicians has done before or after him.'

Paracelsus's ideas were to be expressed in his aphorisms – or, it is safer to say, these aphorisms which were to be attributed to him:

The best of our popular physicians are the ones who do the least harm. But unfortunately some poison their patients with mercury, and others purge or bleed them to death. There are some who have learned so much that their learning has driven out all their common sense, and there are others who care a great deal more for their own profit than for the health of their patients . . .

A physician should be the servant of Nature, not her enemy; he should be able to guide and direct her in her struggle for life, and not throw, by his unreasonable influence, fresh obstacles in the way of recovery.

The knowledge of Nature is the foundation of the science of medicine.

If you wish to be a true physician you must be able to do your own thinking, and not merely employ the thoughts of others.

To be an alchemist is to understand the chemistry of life. Medicine is not merely a science, but an art; it does not consist in compounding pills and plasters and drugs of all kinds, but it deals with the processes of life, which must be understood before they can be guided. A powerful will may cure, where a doubt will end in failure. The character of the physician may act more powerfully upon the patient than all the drugs employed.

The patient must not be out of the physician's mind day and night. He must put his whole power of reasoning and his judgement deliberately in the service of his patient.

Paracelsus – Sigerist concluded in his *Man and Medicine*:

storms the battlements of the four humor theory, the dominant pathology. He makes use of his great medical and scientific experience to create a new theory of disease. To a far greater extent than was true of ancient pathology man, sick and in health, is to him part of the universe, part of the great unchangeable event of nature. His pathology is also natural philosophy, but he often works with theories adopted from the new natural sciences, especially chemistry. Paracelsus remains alone. He is a phenomenon such as may be found at the beginning of a new epoch. He is twofold and great, prophetic and progressive and ahead of his times.

Why, then, has Paracelsus been the target for such abuse? 'He has been held up as the arch-charlatan of history', Osler observed: 'we have taken a cheap estimate of him from Fuller and Bacon, and from a host of scurrilous scribblers who debased or perverted his writings.' Thomas Fuller's *Holy and Profane*

State, published in 1641, showed Paracelsus as exemplifying the drunken quack: 'He was never seen to pray, and seldom came to church. He was not only skilled in natural magic (the utmost bounds whereof border on the suburbs of hell) but is charged to converse constantly with familiars. Guilty he was of all vices but wantonness.' Similar verdicts have been passed by commentators up to the present day: 'a rude, circuitous obscurantist', one of his detractors called him at the time of the fourth centenary of his death 'not a harbinger of light, knowledge and progress'.

Rude, Paracelsus certainly was – a most truculent, opinionated man. Had he acquired humility, he might have had less difficulty in getting his ideas across; but then, had he been more humble, he might not have dared to express them, so at variance were they with the orthodoxy of his time. The real reason why he has continued to be regarded with suspicion is dislike not of his personality but of his cast of mind – revealed in those phrases 'skilled in natural magic' and 'not a harbinger of light'. That Paracelsus should have made an enemy of the Church, holding the views he did, was inevitable (though, contrary to Fuller's assertions, he remained a believer); and though he might be the Luther of medicine, his views were not likely to commend themselves to emergent Protestantism any more than to Rome. But the main reason why obloquy was later poured upon him was that in his own lifetime the process was beginning which was to lead to science hiving off from religion and philosophy. It was a necessary process; but in their anxiety to justify themselves, its exponents were to create what was later to be described as scientism – which may loosely be defined as a quantitative attitude of mind, unconcerned with and usually hostile to all that cannot be measured, analysed and explained; particularly the territory of mysticism and of the occult.

Paracelsus took the opposite view. He observed that there were many phenomena which were inexplicable to man; but he assumed that the fact they were inexplicable made them a suitable subject for study. 'We contain within ourselves', he wrote, 'as many natural powers as heaven and earth possess. Can the magnet draw the iron to itself even though it appears to be a dead thing? . . . Can the climbing vines reach out to the sun? So well may man in similar manner have access to the sun . . . they are all invisible works, and yet they are natural.'

Inevitably, some of his attempts to explain these invisible works sound eccentric today; but it may be premature to jeer at them. The history of science is littered with tales of theories ridiculed as unscientific when they first appeared: Liebnitz contemptuously dismissing Newton's theory of gravitation as occultism: Galileo using the same term to deride Kepler's belief that the moon influences the tides. Many of Paracelsus's hunches were later to be vindicated, or at least shown to be near enough the mark to prove they had been pushing him along the right lines.

Certainly Paracelsus was not a mystic in the sense of being unable to exercise rational discrimination. His belief in the interaction of macrocosm and microcosm did not lead him, as it has lead so many other people, to faith in horoscopes: it couldn't be quite so simple, he thought, as that. 'The wise man can rule and master the stars, and not the stars him . . . a brutish man is ruled, mastered, compelled by the stars, so that he has to follow them like a thief to the gallows.' Quoting this Gregory Zilboorg suggested that 'Paracelsus was almost ready to state that what he actually meant by "the stars" was the sum of the biological influences to which man must succumb when he loses control over things as a result of a weakening of his rational life'. And his attitude to alchemy was very similar. Alchemy, he assumed, was a necessary and valuable type of research, but only when directed to its fundamental aim: it must not be prostituted for personal gain. Its objective should be to make neither gold nor silver, but to understand and master disease.

Alchemists had already acquired the reputation of being interested primarily in the transmutation of baser metals into gold; and obviously this was a lucrative prospect. But the alchemist's real objective was not simply to find a technique to make that change, like a conjuring trick. What they were looking for was something much more fundamental; the source of life and of power. The idea that there was such a source, which might be tapped, appears to have arisen in Egypt, where it had been identified with the mystical body of the God Osiris – a notion appropriated by Christianity to give significance to the sacrament of the Mass. The alchemists, disregarding such interpretations, felt that there must be some source if they could only find it. Pauwels and Bergier quoted a definition of alchemy in their *Le Matin des Magiciens*:

La secret de l'alchemie, le voici; il existe un moyen de manipuler la matière et l'énergie de façon à produire ce que les scientifiques contemporains nommeraient un champ de force. Ce champ de force agit sur l'observateur et le met dans une situation privilegiée en face de l'univers. De ce point privilegiée, il a accés à des realités que l'éspace et le temps, la matière et l'énergie, nous manquent d'habitude.

It follows that the alchemists have been unjustly maligned. Their research may not have been scientific by the standards of their time; but recent discoveries about the nature of nuclear energy, coupled with the acceptance of Heisenberg's principle, show that they were more scientific than orthodoxy was at the time. 'We have entered upon the atomic age', Iago Galdston put it, 'and thus have realised in an egregious fashion the dream of the alchemist.' Pauwels and Bergier went further, arguing that if the writings of the alchemists could once again be studied – this time sympathetically, in the light of recent scientific discoveries – much would be found of far more interest and value than is contained in the great volume of orthodox research, which events have now discredited or rendered irrelevant.

There is no justification, then, for continuing to regard alchemists as unscrupulous charlatans. Sometimes they were: the nature of their occupation and theories, as Ben Jonson noted, was accommodating to fraud

> What's the proper passion of metals?
> Malleation.
> . . . Your *lapis philosophicus*?
> 'Tis a stone,
> And not a stone; a spirit, a soul, and a body:
> Which if you do dissolve, it is dissolved;
> If you coagulate, it is coagulated;
> If you make it fly, it flieth.

And very probably few alchemists appreciated the importance of Paracelsus's fourth pillar, love. Paracelsus turned out to be the last of his line to make an impact on medicine: alchemists, necromancers and magicians continued to operate, but none was to leave any impression until Mesmer, two and a half centuries later.

This is not to say that they were ineffectual as healers. Individuals continued to make local and regional reputations for themselves, with the accoutrements of sorcery; and even at their most absurd, they must often have worked – even down to the 'abracadabra' level. The formula had existed since the reign of the Emperor Caracalla, the usual prescription being that the patient should write out the term, losing one of its letters with each line:

A B R A C A D A B R A
A B R A C A D A B R
A B R A C A D A B
A B R A C A D A
A B R A C A D
A B R A C A
A B R A C
A B R A
A B R
A B
A

With each successive line, the grip of the illness would be relaxed; and if the formula were then worn around the neck as a talisman, it would protect the patient from further trouble. 'Abracadabra' itself has degenerated until it is now the word conjurors use at children's parties, but for centuries it was taken seriously. And that the idea of 'squeezing out' the illness with a formula was not entirely ludicrous was to be surprisingly demonstrated more than 1500 years after its inception, when an experiment was made to compare its efficacy with orthodox treatment, in the removal of warts. Professor Eysenck described the occasion in his *Uses and Abuses of Psychology*:

Two groups of children were used: the control group which received ordinary treatment for their warts; and the experimental group, which was submitted to suggestion treatment. This consisted essentially in drawing a picture of the child's hand, with the wart on it, on a large sheet of paper; and then, with a certain amount of hocus-pocus, drawing circles around the wart and reducing its size on the picture day by day until the wart had completely disappeared in the picture. This procedure, which makes use of suggestibility no less than the famous method used by Tom Sawyer in *Huckleberry Finn*, was shown to be far more effective than the orthodox medical treatment.

If we can assume, as is surely reasonable, that some of the sorcerer's patients in the past were at least as amenable to suggestion as those twentieth-century children, he must often have effected cures – even if sometimes with his tongue in his cheek, and his purse at the ready. To this day in country districts there remain a few practitioners of the art; but the growth of knowledge and of scepticism has pushed sorcery out to a peripheral position in

Opposite: Venetian quacks selling the wonder-drug Theriac

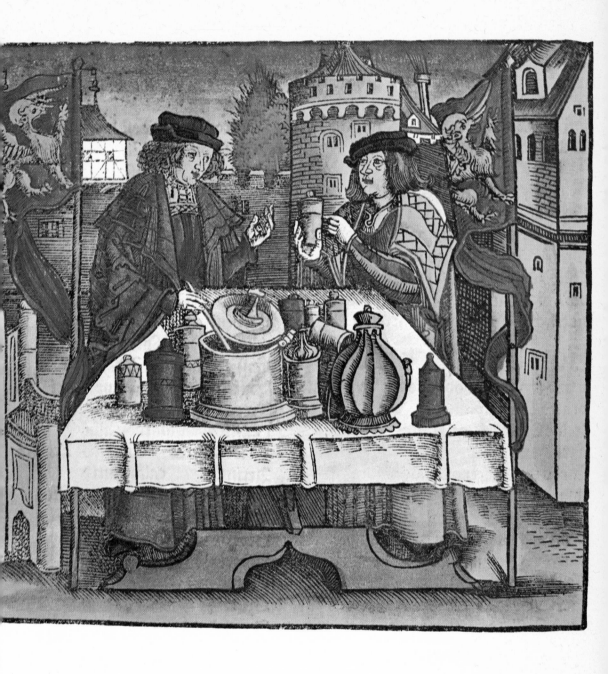

medicine. It lingers on chiefly in the form of occasional medical fads, and in old wives' remedies which sometimes enjoy a fashionable revival.

Vesalius

Paracelsus is not regarded as the central figure of Renaissance medicine; that title is usually given to Andreas Vesalius, born in Brussels in 1514. As a schoolboy, Vesalius had dissected mice, cats and dogs; later, he gratified his curiosity about the workings of the human body by helping to steal the body of a criminal hanged outside the walls of Louvain. But such depredations have never been considered unconventional for medical students; and nothing in Vesalius's early career suggested that he was going to win posterity's acclaim as a rebel – as the iconoclast who thrust open the doors of the dungeon kept barred by centuries' old tradition. The fact that, as a student, he completed a translation of one of the works of Rhazes, and that he was appointed Professor of Surgery and Anatomy at Padua at the age of twenty-three, indicates that he must have given the authorities satisfaction. But his fascination with anatomy led him into dissent; for what he found when he watched the dissection of human bodies, and later dissected them himself, revealed that Galen as an anatomist had been very far from infallible.

That this discovery had not been made long before was due to the prejudice in most parts of the world, and in particular those regions under Christian and Moslem control, against dissection. The Church's edict *Ecclesia abhorret a sanguine*, promulgated in 1163, had been designed to prevent crude operations, but it had amounted to a ban on all but the simplest surgery; and Pope Boniface's *De Sepulturis* decree of 1300 had a similar inhibiting effect on anatomy. Boniface was concerned to stop the practice of boiling the flesh off dead crusaders' bones, in order to send their skeletons back more conveniently and cheaply for burial at home; accordingly, he ordained that 'the practice of this or any similar abuse with regard to the bodies of the dead should cease forever'. There is no evidence that he regarded anatomical dissection as a 'similar abuse' – it was rarely practised; but when interest began to grow in anatomy, the edict was recalled, and invoked – and not simply by the Church: aged teachers of medicine, who for years had relied on the old Galenic illustrations of the human body, were in no mind either to dissect bodies themselves, which they felt would be disgusting, or to have their assumptions challenged by young upstarts. They were relieved to be able to point to the edict, and forbid the practice. In any case, the power of Galen's authority extended even over those who broke or evaded or ignored the ban. Two hundred years before Vesalius's birth, Mundinus of Bologna had managed to get hold of a couple of cadavers and used them for demonstration to students; he wrote a handbook of anatomy, but it revealed the purpose of his dissection had been to prove that Galen and Avicenna had been right.

By the time Vesalius was a student, dissection of the human body had become fairly widespread, and not simply for medical students: Dürer, Michaelangelo and Leonardo da Vinci had all become anatomists, in order to learn more about the human body, its characteristics and its functions – Leonardo arguing in his own defence that those who studied at second-hand through old authors showed themselves to be not the sons, but the stepsons of nature. Even Leonardo at first accepted Galen's anatomy, but his notebooks reveal that experience had demonstrated to him that it was incorrect. Leonardo in fact would now be credited with the first decisive break from the Galen tradition, had his book on anatomy been published; but his indispensable co-worker died, and the project was abandoned.

Vesalius was also originally a Galenist and, like Mundinus, he might conceivably have rationalised his anatomical observations so that they would fit in with Galen's, had inspiration not given him the clue to the cause of the discrepancies. Galen, he realised, had described accurately enough what he was looking at; but what he had been looking at was not human beings, but monkeys and pigs. At once, what had been incomprehensible became simple; and Vesalius set to work and finished his own textbook of anatomy, *De humani corporis fabrica*, published while he was still in his twenties.

Some of the details on which he corrected Galen were of academic interest: it was the fact that a correction had had to be made, and had been published in a manner that allowed for no rebuttal, that mattered. But at this stage the story went sour on Vesalius. Predictably, some traditionalists turned on the newcomer; his own professor in Paris, Sylvius, was to describe him as a 'crazy fool poisoning the air of Europe with his vapourings'. Legend has pictured Vesalius, disillusioned, burning all his notebooks; certainly he left Italy, to become court physician to the King of Spain – living there for another twenty years, in relative obscurity, and dying in 1564 while on a pilgrimage to Jerusalem, reputedly in disgrace.

The standard picture of Vesalius, then, has been of young rebel genius unfairly repudiated by old crusted prejudice. It is an over-simplification. *De humani corporis fabrica* happened to be published less than a week after Copernicus's *De revolutionibus orbium celestium*; and historians of the Renaissance, delighted at this neat coupling, settled on it as a suitable date for the end of an era, and the birth of the new scientific age. But recently both Copernicus and Vesalius have been subjected to more critical scrutiny, and in both cases the legend of the courageous rebel has had to be modified.

Contrary to received opinion, Professor Ashley Montague argued, Vesalius did not regard his book as a break with the Galenical tradition, nor was it so regarded at the time; rather, as an advance upon it. And Sylvius did not, apparently, damn his pupil for substituting observation for tradition – Sylvius had himself been in the habit of urging his students to substitute observation for book-learning – 'reading alone never taught anyone how to sail a ship'. What angered Sylvius was that his pupil should have stolen his thunder, as well as inserting snide remarks about the state of anatomical training. There were a few attacks by bigots on Vesalius, but nothing comparable to the reactionary and inquisitionary rage there would have been a few years earlier, because the foundations of the new anatomy had in fact already been firmly laid by Sylvius and other anatomists – notably by Jacopo da Carpi, of Pavia and Bologna. Carpi had dissected scores of human bodies, and published a commentary of Mundinus which revealed that he, too, was an advocate of observation, rather than reliance on authority; and that he was ready to discard Galen's descriptions whenever his observation showed them to be incorrect.

Vesalius's originality, then, lay not in grasping that Galen had made mistakes: this had been realised, and commented upon, by predecessors. His contribution was to make it clear why Galen had made the mistakes. This was not destructive of the whole Galen edifice – nor was it intended to be. It is still possible to argue, as Ashley Montague did, that 'the name of Galen must continue to be honoured and revered as one of the greatest discoverers and systematisers in the history of biology' and to regard as venial his tendency to extrapolate his findings from animals to human without admitting he had done so. And it was not difficult for medical schools of the period to incorporate Vesalius's work, while continuing to teach Galenism.

There was no question, then, of Galenism being overthrown at a single stroke. A doctor who was seeking membership of the English College of Physicians in 1560 could still be told that he would be admitted, 'but not until he had signed a recantation of his error in having impugned the infallibility of Galen'; and in university courses, Galen, Avicenna and the rest continued to be staple until the end of the century. When they disappeared, it was not so much because rebels had driven them out by force of argument, but because they had ceased to be relevant. Vesalius was part of this process, because his book appeared in time to catch the tide; but he did not cause the tide to flow, and he is less a representative Renaissance figure than his more congenial contemporary, Paré.

Paré

Of the figures who dominate the Renaissance medical scene, much the most agreeable is Ambroise Paré. Paracelsus was an egomaniac, and Vesalius for no very clear reason unlikable; but Paré not merely did much to raise the status of his branch of the profession, he did it modestly and endearingly.

Until his time, surgery in Europe had been of little account. In India at the time of Susruta the surgeon had been a respected figure, as Albucasis had helped to make him in Spain; but this was unusual. Avicenna considered surgery should not be regarded as on the same level as general medical practice: and in medieval Europe, apart from the Church's objections, there was a general feeling that it was a subject with which the medical student ought not to concern himself: some schools formally banned it. Surgeons, in fact, held much the same status as chiropractors today – but with none of the mystique the chiropractor sometimes breeds among his patients.

Ordinarily, the surgeon was a barber: his operations were done 'on the side' (much as blacksmiths until recently often used to double as bonesetters in country districts). He did not as a rule perform operations in the modern sense of the term: he was there to assist in bleedings, in pulling teeth, in lancing abscesses, and in making the occasional emergency amputation. There were educated specialist surgeons in Christian Europe in medieval times, but they were the exception until in the thirteenth century Henri de Mondeville and a handful of others began to establish surgery as a craft in its own right; and they did not win recognition until Guy de Chauliac became physician to Pope Clement VI. Guy's *Chirurgia Magna* was not an original work, being largely based on Albucasis; nor was it particularly enlightened; but the fact that a man of his learning and influence should have written a book on surgery at all was significant.

One of Guy's complaints about surgery at the time was that its practitioners were 'surgeons of the short robe' – barbers. By this time, in the opinion of the surgeons of the long robe – qualified doctors who undertook surgery – the barbers were getting above themselves, and performing operations for gallstones, hernias, and even for cataract. A class division arose, clinically demarcated by the surgeons, whenever they could, with the help of restrictive practices – such as refusing to allow the barbers to treat patients in hospitals. The physicians held aloof from this contest, regarding both surgeons and barbers as of small account.

Paré was a country boy, of no formal education, who had been a barber's apprentice; but somehow he managed to wangle his way into the Hôtel Dieu in Paris and gain experience there before joining the French army as a regimental surgeon – an occupation for which the invention of gunpowder had greatly increased the demand. A single explosion might burn and wound scores of men, all of whom had to be treated; if the surgeon was able to restore them quickly to the ranks it mattered little to his commanders that his academic qualifications might be slender. And from the first, Paré showed himself exceptionally good at his job.

He is best known for the experiment by which he revealed the inadequacy of the standard method of treating gunshot wounds. It had been assumed that these wounds were poisoned by the gunpowder, and that they must therefore be cauterised with a mixture of boiling oil and treacle. Paré was revolted by this method because of the pain it caused; but finding that every military surgeon used it, he felt bound to do the same. Then:

It chanced one time, that because of the great numbers wounded I ran out of oil. A few remained to be dressed; and rather than seem to do nothing for them I applied a lotion of yolk of egg, oil of roses, and turpentine. I could not sleep all that night for worry, as the dressing disturbed my thoughts; I feared the next day I should find them dead, or on the point of death, from the poison in their wounds which I had not dressed with boiling oil. So I got up early to visit my patients – and unexpectedly, I found that those I had dressed with the lotion not only had suffered no severe pain, and had a good night's rest; their wounds were not even inflamed. But the others, who had been burned with the boiling oil, were feverish and in

85

agony; and the flesh around their wounds was swollen. And when I had many times tried this in other cases I decided that neither I nor anybody else should ever cauterise a gunshot wound again.

Needless to say, the surgeons of the long robe thought Paré presumptuous: the medical faculty in Paris actually petitioned the city authorities not to allow his writings, 'the works of a very impudent and ignorant fellow', to be sold without the faculty's approval. They were furious with Paré not simply because he was telling them that what had been standard treatment for years was wrong: what worried them more was that he wrote in the vernacular, so that their errors would be exposed to the public. Nor were they at all appeased by Paré's humility, which made him repeat, when praised for a patient's recovery, 'I treated him: God cured him'; this suggested all too low an opinion of the power of the doctor. But Paré's fame as a surgeon continued to spread; he was appointed surgeon-in-ordinary to the court: and eventually he had grudgingly to be admitted into the fraternity of the long robe – even without Latin.

What was particularly endearing about Paré was his resolute refusal to accept current medical fashion as gospel. He liked tried remedies, but he wanted them to be tested, as well; and he was continually experimenting with old-wives'-tale cures, not to discredit them, but to see whether there might be truth in them. It is risky with Paré – who gaily appropriated the ideas of others whenever he liked them – to be sure he was not romancing in retrospect; but some of the episodes he recounts, or are attributed to him, are too amiable to be rejected – particularly the story of his test of an old crone's remedy for burns: raw chopped onion. Paré had the inspiration of treating, with the raw chopped onion, one cheek of a German soldier whose face had been burned, the other cheek, with his own standard cooling lotion. He found, as further tests were to verify, that the onion was more efficacious. He did not, admittedly, succeed in convincing later generations of surgeons that onion was the best remedy (to this day argument continues within the profession which remedies *are* best for burns; it is not without interest that an eminent medical journal recently carried an article setting forth convincingly the claims of milk). But the value of Paré's experiments was that they were not inhibited by prejudice. He refused to reject remedies because they were too simple, or because they sounded ridiculous. And his aim was always to relieve suffering; not to gain kudos for himself.

Paré was not the only surgeon of his era to win a reputation. In the later part of the century Gaspare Tagliacozzi revived the operation of rhinoplasty, which Indian surgeons had perfected many centuries before: transplanting a flap of skin from the patient's arm, which was kept bandaged to the head until the graft had caught on and formed a new nose (particularly useful to men who had their noses cut off for some offence). But although this and other operations were developed after Paré's death, there is a sense in which it can be said that Paré took surgery almost as far as it could go, so long as anaesthetics and asepsis were lacking. Until these allies were enlisted, improvements could only be marginal. There was still room for new theories of surgery to develop, on the basis of Vesalius's anatomy; in the eighteenth century John Hunter, for one, did much to make it more scientific. But in the art of surgery, Paré was to represent the peak of achievement for centuries.

Epidemics

The bubonic plague had become endemic in Europe after the Black Death, reappearing sporadically with something like its original violence, though not again so widespread; but the Renaissance also was ushered in by other varieties of epidemic, less destructive but occasionally even more alarming in their unpredictability – as in the case of the sweating sickness, a particularly violent type of influenza. Britain was the worst sufferer, a fact that was attributed to the weather.

Opinions differ about the date of the first visitation, but Hecker dramatically linked it to the Battle of Bosworth, on August 22, 1485, when Richard III lost his life and his throne.

The joy of the nation was clouded by a mortal disease which thinned the ranks of the warriors, and following in the rear of Henry's victorious army, spread in a few weeks from the distant mountains of Wales to the metropolis of the empire. It was a violent inflammatory fever which, after a short rigor, prostrated the powers as with a blow; and amidst painful oppression at the stomach, head-ache, and lethargic stupor, suffused the whole body with a fetid perspiration. All this took place in the course of a few hours, and the crisis was always over within the space of a day and a night.

Two Lord Mayors and six Aldermen died within a week of celebrating their new king's arrival; and his coronation had to be postponed.

Those who still clung to the Christian belief that epidemics were a form of divine retribution for the wickedness of mankind were given what they could regard as striking confirmation when a new – or so it seemed – epidemic struck in Europe just before the end of the fifteenth century: syphilis, which broke out in Naples after its capture by the French in 1495. The Neapolitans, assuming the invaders must have brought it with them, called it the French disease; the French, assuming that they had picked it up at their destination, called it Neapolitan. But on reflection, the blame was soon put on Columbus and his followers, who had returned from the New World in 1494, and who could therefore be presumed to have brought it back with them. This explanation has been disputed on the grounds that the disease spread too fast too far to be thus accounted for; but it would fit in with the common pattern of epidemics – arising because the virus is exported from a region where it has been only mildly painful, or even harmless to man, to another region where the local population have not acquired immunity, and suffer severely in consequence. Certainly when it first broke out in Europe, as described by Fracastoro (who gave it the name syphilis) the symptoms were hideous. Fracastoro chose to relate them in verse:

> Soon is the body ulcerous and vile.
> The face becomes, within a little while,
> A mask of running pustules, small and great
> A horny shell that glands will irritate
> Breaking, and emptying an acrid humor
> From pus-corroded skin pours every tumor.
> And bloody ulcers deeply dig away
> Granwing the tissues that they make their prey
> Then is man stripped until his piteous moans
> Come from a skeleton of putrid bones.

This was written in 1530; but by the time Fracastoro's *De Contagione* appeared in 1546, he could confidently claim that the symptoms of the disease, though still unpleasant, were far less loathsome than they had been earlier.

Unlike most works of its kind, *De Contagione* was hailed by contemporaries

The Renaissance.

At an anatomy lesson at Padua in the fifteenth century, the lecturer is assisted by a
dissector and a demonstrator

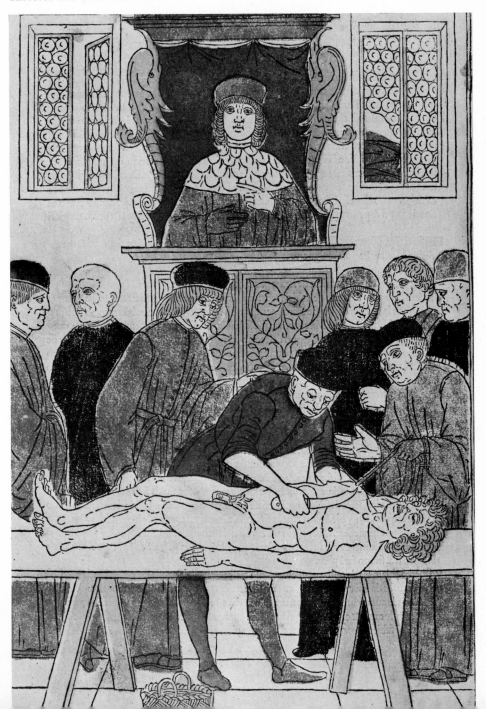

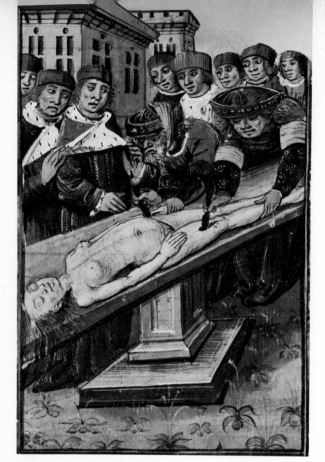

Anatomical dissection in the Middle Ages, attended by knights

Dissection with five surgeons. From the head of the chapter on 'Man' in the *Proprietaire des Choses* (1482)

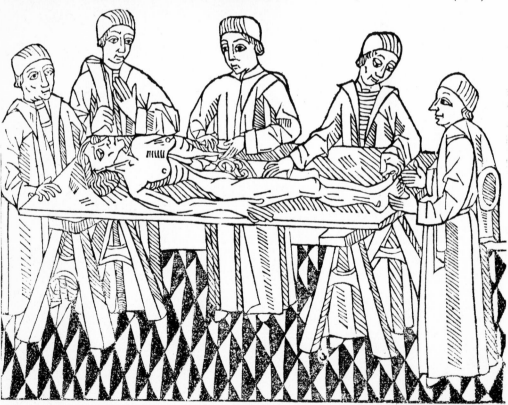

This skeleton (1493) by Richard Hela of Nuremberg presents a remarkable advance on the purely schematic diagrams of the Middle Ages

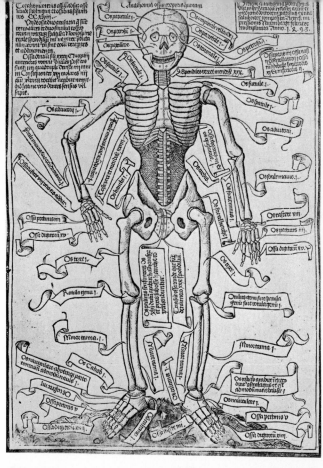

Leonardo da Vinci's drawing of the 'Tree of the Vessels'. Leonardo's studies disproved Galen's theories of the blood-system, but his work was not published

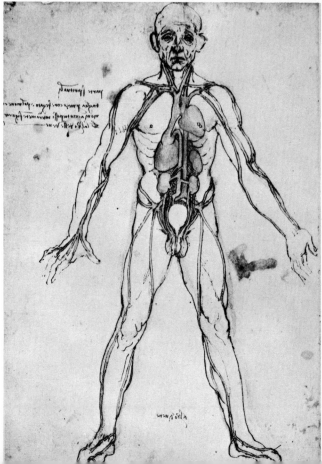

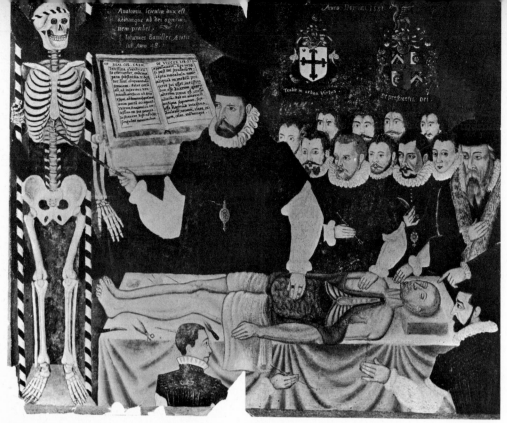

The London barber-surgeon John Banister, giving an anatomy lesson, points simultaneously to the skeleton and to the dissected corpse

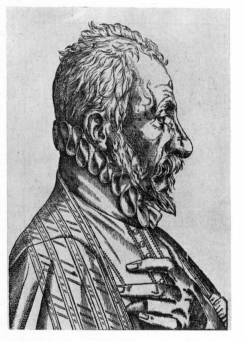

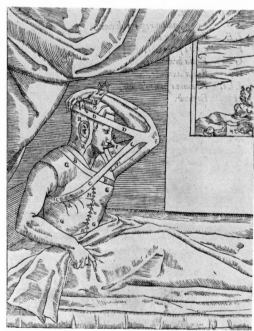

Left: The surgeon Ambroise Paré at the age of 65. From the second edition (1579) of his works

Right: Skin-grafting in the sixteenth century. From Tagliacozzi's *De Curtorum Chirurgia*

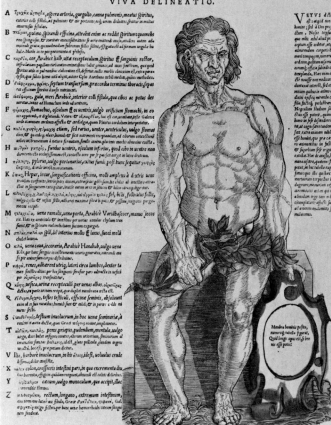

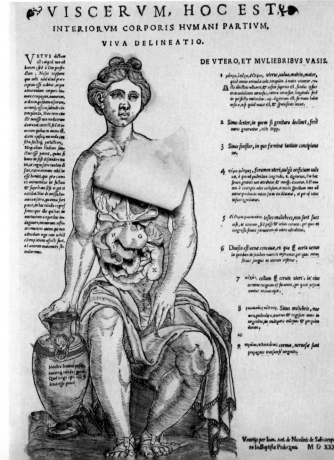

Adam and Eve with folding flaps revealing all the internal organs; based on Vesalius' principles of anatomy and probably from drawings by Vesalius himself

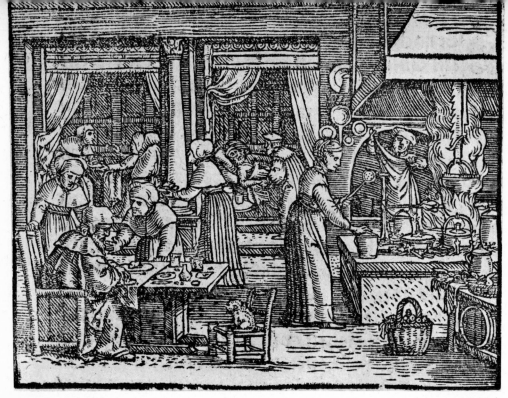

Paracelsus' regulations for the sick insisted that they should be made to rest and given a healthy and varied diet. 'Good medicine with bad care and good care with bad medicine are equally useless'

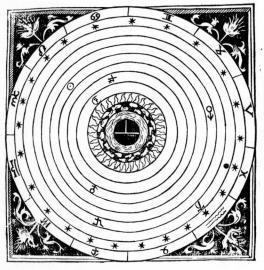

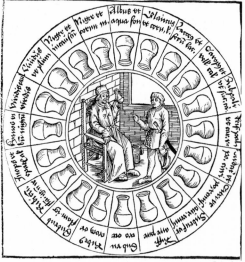

Left: Illustration to Paracelsus' theories of celestial effects on the healing of wounds

Right: The mainstay of the Renaissance physician was still the examination of urine. The table shows the significance of the colour of urine

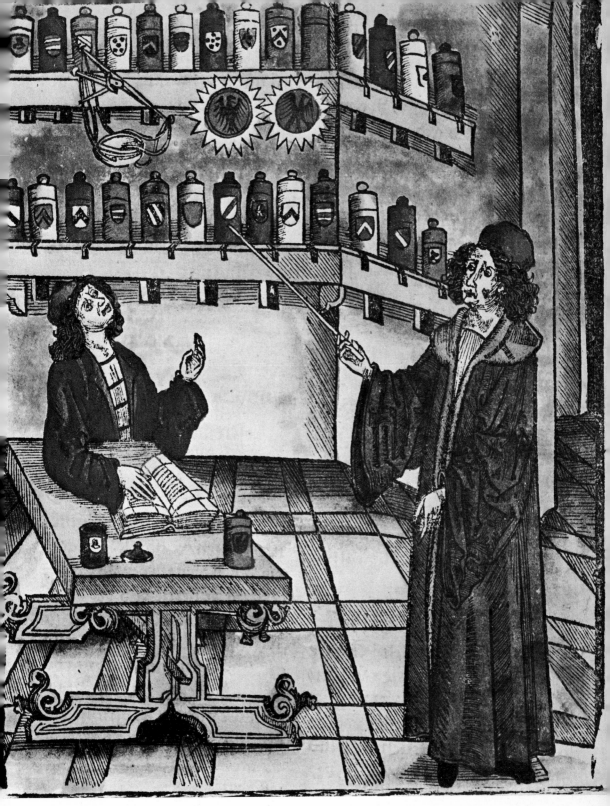

A doctor orders a preparation to be made up by the apothecary, who consults his herbal

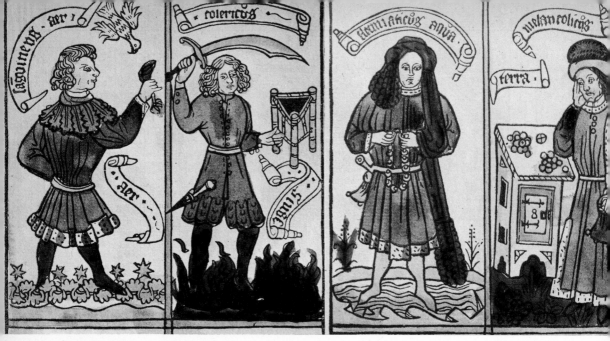

Medical theory still leaned heavily on the idea of the four temperaments, sanguine, choleric, phlegmatic and melancholy; associated with air, fire, water and earth

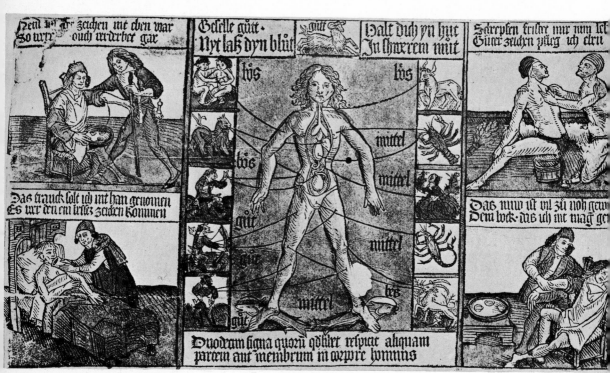

Calendar showing the seasons propitious for blood-letting. The scenes at the side show bleeding, cupping in the bath-house, administering medicine and feeling the pulse

as a notable achievement – as it was; the first comprehensive explanation of how infectious diseases spread: by direct contact; by indirect contact, as through clothing; and through the air. Fracastoro also revived the Hippocratic notion of observing symptoms the better to differentiate one variety of disease from another. He deserves his place, then, in the gallery of the medical figures of the Renaissance; but chiefly as a cataloguer, not as a doctor. He preferred to study epidemics from the seclusion of his elegant country home; and though the fame his books won him led to his being appointed official physician to the Council of Trent, his stay at that protracted assembly was extremely brief.

The fact was that Fracastoro had nothing new to offer in the way of treatment of syphilis or any other disorder. He recounted various remedies that had been recommended and tried out, but he held out no great hopes for them; falling back on Paracelsus's prescription, mercury ointment, which was to continue to feature, rather despairingly, in the treatment of the pox for centuries. And in spite of the high regard in which Fracastoro's work was held, its implications were not grasped. Early in the fifteenth century the Venetian republic, which had enjoyed the advice of a small public health department for over fifty years, decided that one effective measure against epidemics would be to isolate arrivals from plague areas. The system worked; other ports began to adopt it; and eventually the Marseilles' rule, insisting upon forty days' isolation for arrivals, became accepted and passed into the language as quarantine. But there, inventiveness ceased. It did not occur to local or regional authorities that if these epidemics could not be stopped it was all the more important to seek fresh ways to prevent them from breaking out – say, by making arrangements to seal off plague-affected areas, and introducing better sanitation and hygiene.

The degree of official helplessness becomes even more curious in connection with the other great contagion that was to become endemic in Europe in this period: typhus. By a coincidence, it was at Naples that typhus struck its first decisive blow; and this time, in 1528, the French troops were again the besiegers. By midsummer the defenders were just about ready to surrender. Then, typhus broke out in the French camp; within a month well over half the army was dead; the siege of Naples had to be raised; and what remained of the French army quickly disintegrated.

The consequences of that outbreak, Zinsser thought, were incalculable.

Had Naples fallen, the Pope would have gone over to the French – with all that that would have meant. As it was, the Emperor triumphed; Italy became dependent upon Spain, and the Papacy on the Emperor; and 'in 1530 Charles V was crowned ruler of the Roman Empire at Bologna, by the power of typhus fever'. And from this time typhus acquired an astonishing ascendancy over the armies and sometimes the navies of the European powers. Yet such was the blindness of kings and governments that they simply refused to recognise its significance; little or nothing was done to examine ways to avoid losing men by it, in spite of the formidable losses due to outbreaks, and their effect on manpower, always chronically short. Generals continued to behave as if it was their military genius alone which decided the issue of a campaign; again and again they neglected elementary precautions which could have been decisive in controlling, if not banishing, epidemics and giving them victory instead of defeat. Most historians, Zinsser complained, have accepted this, referring to the impact of disease only in passing – if at all – as if it was something outside the general's control. Yet, 'other things being approximately equal, that army will win which has the best engineering and sanitary services. The wise general will do what his engineering and sanitary officers tell him. The only reason why this is not entirely apparent in wars is because the military minds on both sides are too superb to notice that both armies are simultaneously immobilised by the same disease.'

In the sixteenth century, however, it would have availed a general little to listen to his sanitary officers, even if his establishment had allowed for them. They would not have known what to recommend. The members of the medical profession, baffled, simply shrugged off infectious diseases as not their concern. Thomas Linacre, who attended Henry VIII and was the founder of the College of Physicians, had plenty of experience of the sweating sickness, but it did not occur to him to work on it: such disorders were outside his clinical terms of reference.

In medieval times, people had at least had some grounds for hope. They could be buoyed up by belief either in an amulet, or in the infinite mercy of God. By the sixteenth century these consolations were no longer so commonly available. Sorcery was still losing ground, presumably because it was so obviously ineffective against epidemic disease; and the Christian attitude to God's part in the proceedings was undergoing yet another change. Christians were no longer accepting, as Boccaccio had done, the proposition that mankind as a whole might have brought punishment on itself by its wickedness. The spread of militant Protestantism, and the militant Catholic reaction to it, was destructive of humility; the leaders of the various sects simply could not allow themselves, let alone their followers, to believe that God would have inflicted such a punishment on his elect. Instead, they assumed that a plague must be the work of the devil, through his human agents: heretics, Jews or witches.

The type of mental derangement which we associate with the term 'witch-hunting' appears to have been a disorder arising from the same source as the dancing mania, which in the sixteenth century began to decline. The dancing mania, on this admittedly over-simplified thesis, had represented a simple release mechanism, whereby people threw off the intolerable unconscious guilt feelings that possessed them. Now a more sophisticated form of release was provided: the guilt could be transferred to witches.

That active witch-hunters are the victims of a form of paranoia (where they are not, as in Senator McCarthy's case, cynically exploiting human gullibility for political ends) is generally accepted; but because the curious paraphernalia of witchcraft – spell-weaving, crones riding on broomsticks by moonlight – has been discarded as superstition, the idea that people actually were bewitched has tended to go into discard, too. But it frequently happened, and on an epidemic scale.

The precise workings of hysteria have still to be clarified; but its symptoms, from the paralysis of Breuer's 'Anna O' to the stigmata of the saintly, have long since been abstracted from the arcane. They can be categorised and labelled, even if not yet fully explained; there is no difficulty in interpreting witchcraft in terms of mental disorder. Its symptoms have even been given impressive-sounding names; thus, the tell-tale marks left by succubi have been classified as 'hysteric ecchymoses'.

Under certain conditions, people in a group in which a strong emotional charge has been generated are released from their normal controls and inhibitions; they go into convulsions: sometimes emotional, sometimes physical, sometimes both. In such circumstances, there is ordinarily a strong element of what appears to be imitativeness – in that individuals are all doing, or saying, much the same sort of thing; but is not calculated imitation. There is no question of follow-my-leader: sometimes members of the group may be performing the same actions out of sight of one another. They are the victims of some corporate force: some emotional contagion.

'Sympathetic' illness, as it has been called, is well known in hospitals; on a small scale it is almost an everyday occurrence, with patients collecting symptoms from each other. Sometimes it can be dramatic, as in the outbreak at the Royal Free Hospital in London in 1955, where nurses and doctors (but not patients) collapsed with a nervous disorder, a kind of mock polio, with spasms – fortunately not fatal, but hard to shake off; and such outbreaks have been reported from many parts of the world. In them, people behave oddly, and out of character; yet their symptoms often conform to an established pattern. Where in medieval times the disorder was linked with diabolic possession, victims frequently acted and talked as if possessed by whatever happened to be their society's conventional notion of the devil. When they described how they had been bewitched, they were not necessarily lying – though often they were, to implicate an enemy or to escape torture. Sometimes they *had* been – but not by a witch. They were suffering from the prevailing epidemic of hysteria: and the form it took mimicked what were assumed to be the results of witchcraft. Thus, the inmates of monasteries might be afflicted with a disorder that made them mew like cats – cats being associated with witches. In other outbreaks the nuns went into grotesque indecent spasms (as in the Loudun affair); or shouted obscenities while under the influence of the disease. They were not acting their parts, on the instructions of an inquisitor: they were deranged.

Sir Kenelm Digby, a member of the first council of the Royal Society, had an interesting explanation:

I could make a notable recital of such passions that happened to the nuns at Loudun; but having done it in a particular discourse at my return from that Country, where as exactly as I could I discussed the point, I will forbear speaking thereof at this time, otherwise then to pray you to remember, that when two Lutes, or two Harps, near one another, both set to the same tune, if you touch the strings of the one, the other consonant harp will sound at the same time, though no body touch it; whereof Galileo hath ingeniously rendered the reason.

But the fact that diabolic possession is the symptom of an epidemic disease, and a common one (much commoner to this day than is generally realised) was not understood: nor would people have accepted it had it been put forward. As Freud was later to demonstrate, neurosis arises as a protection from an uglier reality; and belief in witchcraft was the neurosis of the age of Enlightenment: one of many indications that emergence of more rational attitudes was capable of creating grave emotional disturbances, because the demands of the unconscious were not being satisfied. In particular there was guilt over the new sexual freedom. In his *History of Medical Psychology* Zilboorg noted the anti-erotic and misogynous nature of the witch-hunting of this period: particularly from the authors of the *Malleus Maleficarum*, published in 1487. The role of sex in our civilisation, he suggested, and man's attitude to woman's place in social life

is thrown into painful relief in this piece of legalistic and theological literature of the early Renaissance. The Old World seems to have risen against woman and written this gruesome testimonial to its own madness ... Never in the history of humanity was woman more systematically degraded. She paid for the fall of Eve seven-fold, and the Law bore a countenance of pride and self-satisfaction and the delusional certainty that the will of the Lord had been done.

As with other forms of epidemic, the medical profession – by this time beginning to be recognisably such, with physicians, surgeons and apothecaries (who were then closer to the modern general practitioner than to the modern chemist) trying to establish themselves with charters of rights and privileges – turned its back on mental disorders, deciding they were none of its concern.

Only a few doctors cared to go against the tide, and insist that mental disorder ought to be their business; and they were ignored. Nevertheless two of them command respect, though their names are all but forgotten. Juan Luis Vives, born in Valencia in 1592, became the friend and counsellor of Catherine of Aragon, moving to London in her service, and winning the respect of Thomas More and of Erasmus. He was not a doctor; in fact he is best remembered in Britain for his elegant prayers, some of which found their way into the official Elizabethan Private Prayer Book – though he remained a Catholic. Disillusioned with Henry VIII, he eventually settled in Bruges; and among his writings was one which reflected his humanism, revolted at the treatment of the mentally afflicted. They should, he urged, be treated as patients:

Some need medical care and attention to their mode of life; others need gentle and friendly treatment, so that like wild animals they may gradually grow gentle; still others require force and chains, but these must be so used that the patients are not made more violent. Above all, as far as possible, tranquillity must be introduced in their minds, for it is through this that reason and sanity return.

Today, when this thesis is generally accepted (though far from universally obeyed) it is difficult to realise what a revolution in thought it represented. Vives and his contemporary, Paracelsus, were committing what could easily be punished as blasphemy. And how unsafe that era was for medical free-thinkers was soon to be shown by the fate of the Spaniard Michael Servetus, Vesalius's fellow-pupil, whose explanation of the way that the blood circulates, though not entirely correct, contradicted Galen and pointed the way for Harvey a century later. Servetus's circulation theory, however, did not attract as much attention at the time as his earlier treatise on prescribing, in which he earned the affection of posterity by suggesting ways to make unpleasant drugs more palatable – by sugaring the pill. This had helped to make him known; and when he went on to his speculations on blood, and in particular on its relationship to the Holy Spirit, his ideas excited the resentment of the authorities, Protestant as well as Catholic. The Inquisition condemned him to death; but it was the sadistic Calvin who trapped him and sent him to the stake. Vives himself remained an orthodox member of his Church; but that might not have been a sufficient safeguard against inquisitors. Had he lived elsewhere, he might have suffered for his repudiation of the belief that insanity was a sign of God's wrath or of the devil's occupation.

Servetus is remembered: but scores of doctors must have been sent to their death because of their religion whose fate is not recorded. Jewish doctors, in particular, were perpetually in danger owing to the possibility that an outbreak of an epidemic might be attributed to their machinations; they were forbidden to practise by successive Popes in the second half of the sixteenth century, and banned from studying medicine at European universities. What they might have contributed to medicine can only be estimated from what Jewish doctors eventually did contribute, when they gained full civil rights in the nineteenth century; but until then – although a few individuals flourished as (in one historian's description) 'a sort of contraband luxury' whose services independent-minded princes liked to enjoy at court – they were prevented from making any significant contribution.

Vives's ideas were expanded by Jonathan Weyer. Born in Holland, Weyer worked and wrote in a German state where the duke who was his patron gave him freedom not only to pursue his interest in mental disorders, but to write freely about them. His best known case history concerned a girl popularly believed to be capable of living indefinitely without food. Weyer, though certain that she was cheating, did not approach the case in the spirit of a prosecuting attorney: he broke down the girl's defences not by cunning but by kindness and sympathy; cured her; and took care to protect her from the wrath of the gullible authorities when they found that they had been deceeived. To Weyer, sufferers from mental disorder, psychotic, neurotic or psychopathic, needed such sympathetic treatment – including witches, and those possessed by devils. His *De Praestigiis Daemonum*, published in the vernacular in 1567, was a comprehensive and courageous demolition of *Malleus Malleficarum*. There might be people, he conceded, who used their powers for wicked ends; but the great majority of 'witches' were simply sick, and should be treated as patients – if anyone should be treated as criminal, it should be their torturers.

To Weyer, Zilboorg argued:

a psychological fact was a fact to be understood and not a phenomenon by which to be aroused, or which should be approved or condemned . . . He was the first clinical and the first descriptive psychiatrist to leave to succeeding generations a heritage which was accepted, developed and perfected into an observational branch of medicine . . . more than anybody else he completed, or at least brought closer to completion, the process of divorcing medical psychology from theology, and empirical knowledge of the human mind from the faith in the perfection of the human soul . . . in the light of these considerations the fervent, revolutionary humanism of Weyer stands out as a phenomenon which must be assessed not merely as a striking episode in medical history, but as a momentous step in the whole history of man.

But Weyer's ideas sank without trace at the time; and for all Zilboorg's impassioned – and justified – eulogy, his name is rarely bracketed with the great innovators in medical history – or even with the supporting cast. The assiduous Garrison refers to him in passing; in most other standard medical histories in the English language, even his name does not appear.

8

THE SEVENTEENTH CENTURY

Science and Sydenham

IN some respects, then, the Renaissance may have been an age of enlighten-ment: in medicine it was a dark age. The genius of such men as Paracelsus, Paré and Weyer illuminated it for posterity, but not for contemporaries, who continued to cling to a delapidated Galenism inadequately propped up by sorcery, astrology and religion. And the seventeenth century, though its reputation stands higher because of the stirrings of scientific curiosity, was little improvement: not, at least, from the patient's point of view.

The prescriptions made out by doctors of the era often resemble those which had been common in the more degenerate days of Ancient Egypt. Bile, dung, ground-up sexual organs, urine, and sweat feature prominently, sometimes with the injunction that they should be taken according to the astrological indications. The most eminent scientists of the time still had no hesitation in accepting the significance of occult influences. Robert Boyle sug-gested powdered mistletoe as a remedy for the falling sickness, 'as much as will lie upon a sixpence, early in the morning, in black cherry water, for some days near the full moon'; and in Paris, Louis XIV's physician asserted that a proper understanding of astrology was a *sine qua non* for medical practice.

Techniques of a magico-religious origin abounded. The best known was 'touching' for the 'King's Evil' – scrofula, a tubercular disorder of the glands of the neck. It had been known from the time of Edward the Con-fessor, but in the seventeenth century it began to become a standard chore of royal life, until rejected by cynical William of Orange, who according to legend 'touched' only one victim, remarking 'may God give you better health and more sense' (Queen Anne was to revive the custom, Samuel Johnson being one of the beneficiaries).

The Seventeenth Century

Henry IV of France (1553–1610) touching for King's Evil

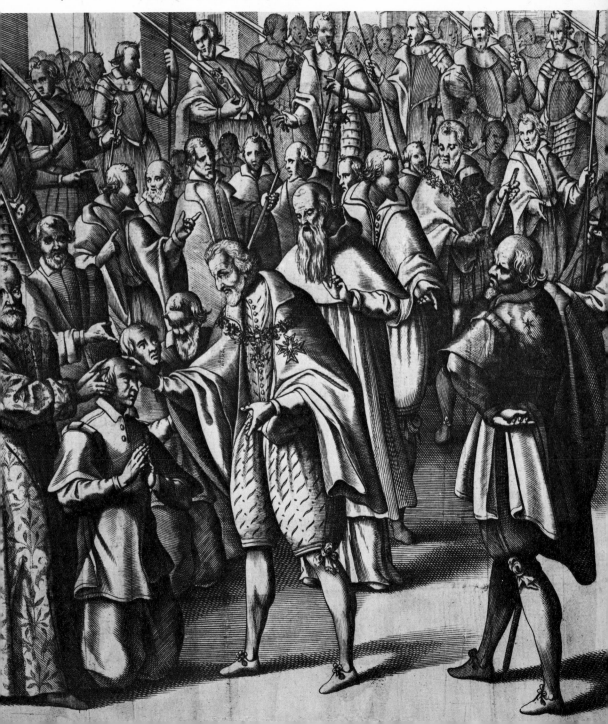

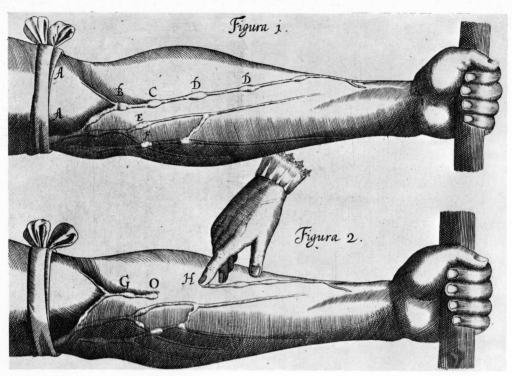

Figura 1.

Figura 2.

Illustration from the first edition of Harvey's *De Motu Cordis* (1628), showing how blood in veins and arteries can flow in only one direction

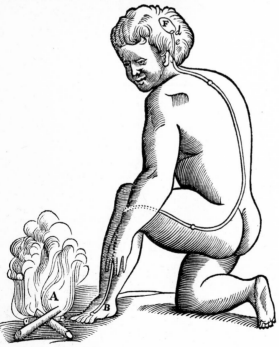

The approach of the iatrophysicists is exemplified by Descartes' theory of perception. The figure illustrates his theories on the nervous system

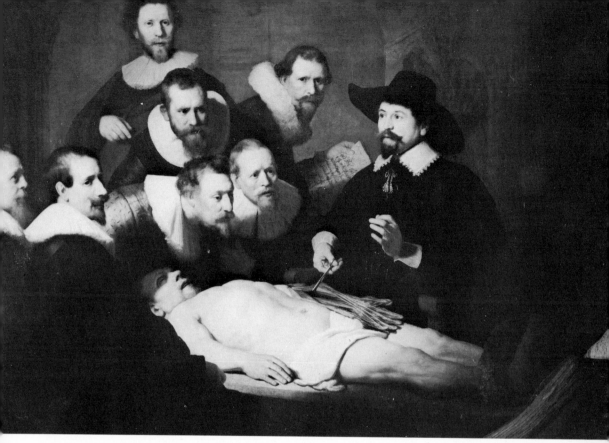

Rembrandt's painting of *Dr Tulp's Anatomy Lesson* (1632)

The anatomical theatre at Leiden, built on the pattern of the famous sixteenth-century theatre at Padua

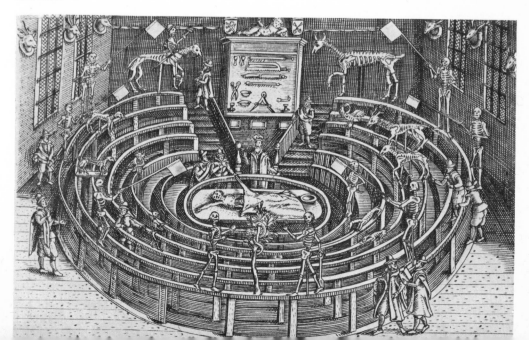

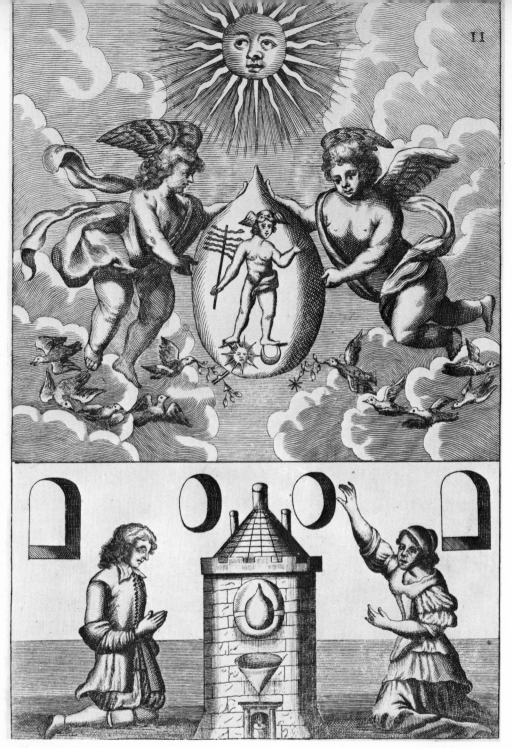

Alchemy continued to influence developments in medicine, particularly the work of the iatrochemists. The plate illustrates the mystical union of sun and moon in the vessel of Hermes. The two alchemists pray by their furnace that the union will take place

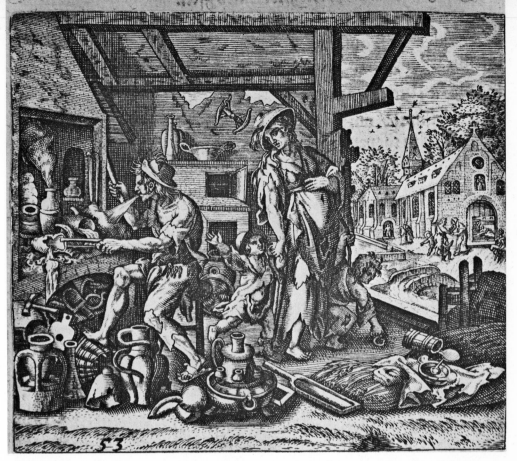

The popular image of the alchemist; a man obsessed with the desire to make gold, while reducing himself, his wife and children to poverty

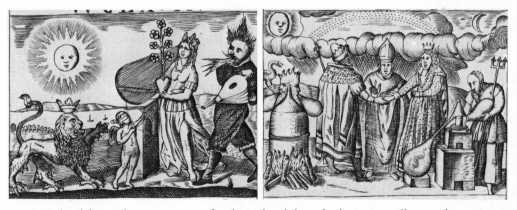

Stages in the alchemist's *magnum opus* of making the philosopher's stone are illustrated emblematically in the *Twelve Keys* of Basil Valentine; two are shown here

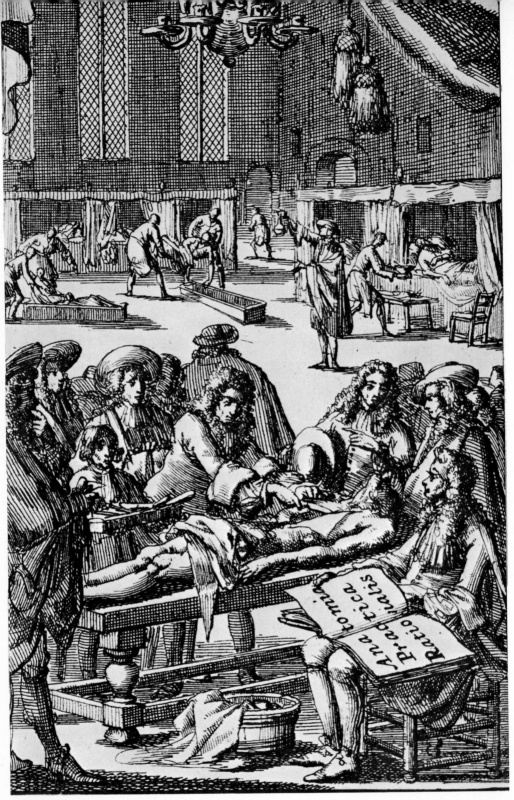

Title-page of a book on anatomy. Even when the dissection of corpses was not actually carried out in a hospital ward, doctors would often go straight to the wards from the dissecting room

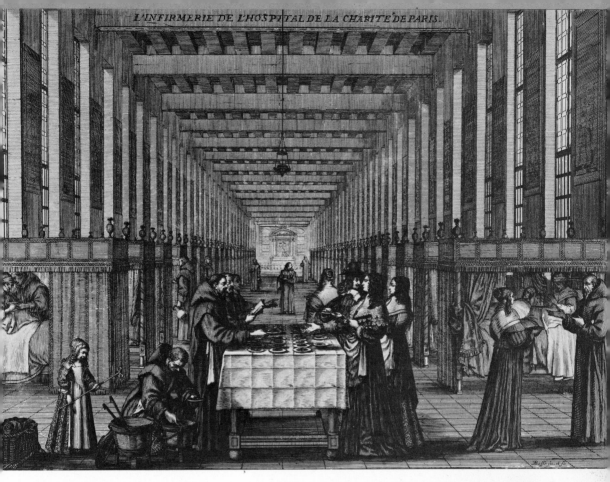

From the Middle Ages onwards
many of the hospitals were run by
monks. Abraham Bosse's engraving
shows the Hôpital de la Charité in
Paris

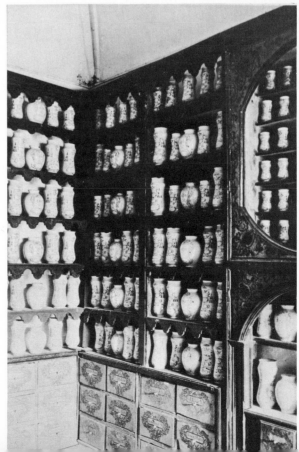

Pharmacies were also found in
many monasteries, as at Santo
Domingo de Silos in Spain

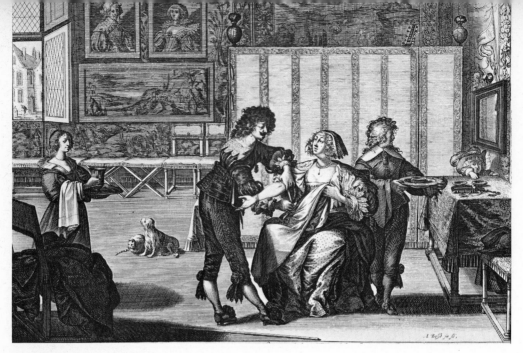

Blood-letting was still normal practice. Bosse's engraving shows a surgeon attending a fashionable lady

Molière not merely satirized both doctor and hypochondriac in his plays; he actually appeared as both: as M. de Porceaugnac with a gigantic syringe and as Argan, *le malade imaginaire*

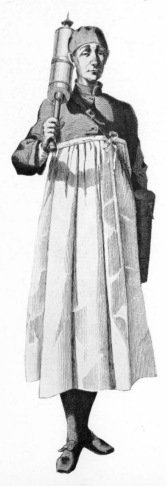

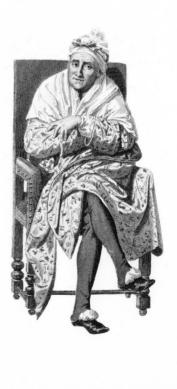

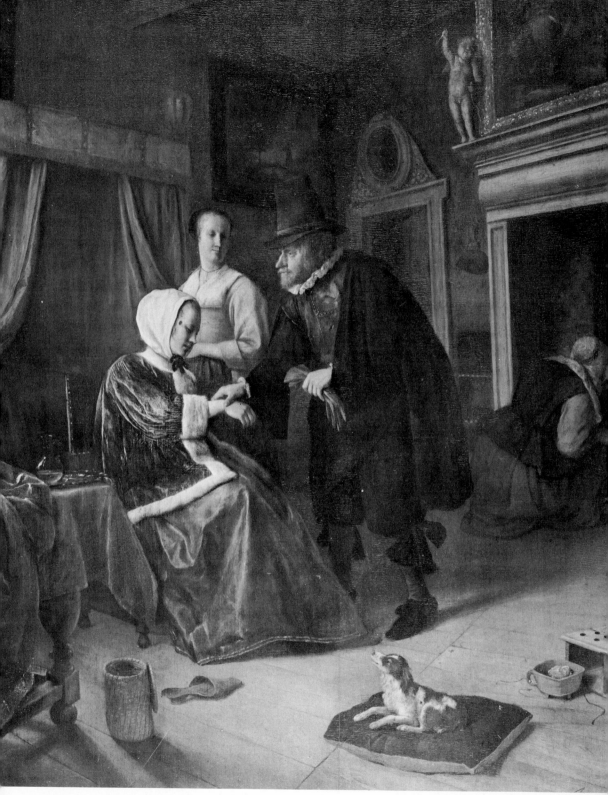

The Love-sick Girl, by Jan Steen — a popular ailment, as Molière's plays and the many pictures depicting the subject show

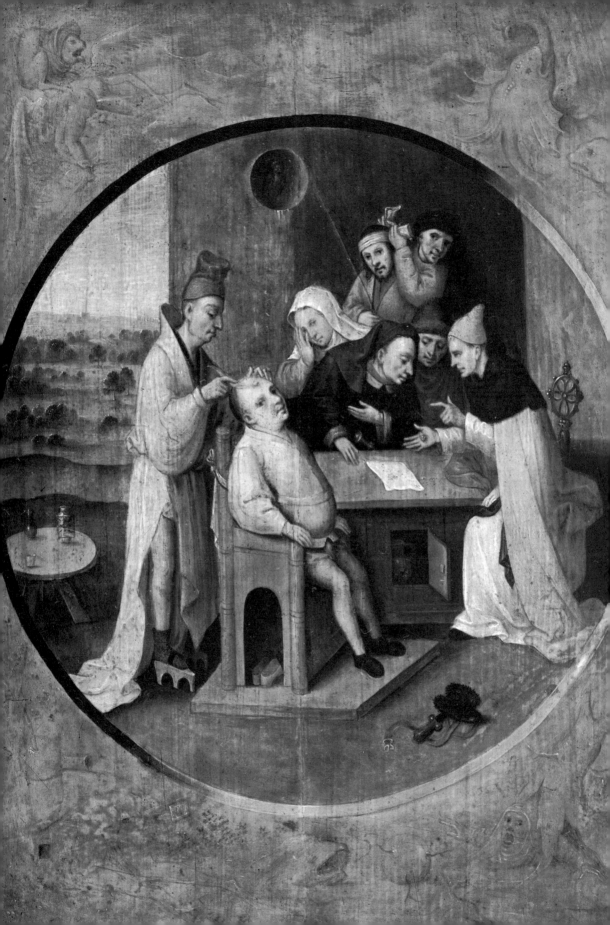

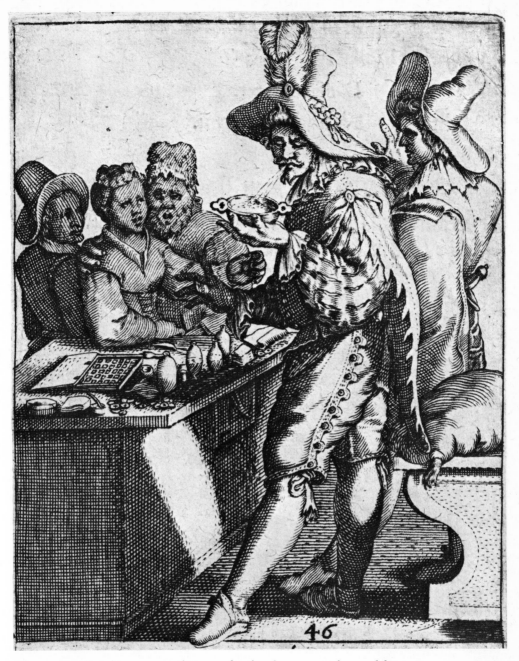

46

The quack, selling his patent medicines, a familiar figure at markets and fairs

Left: A 'stone-cutter' by Jerome Bosch. In the Low Countries these travelling specialists were popular throughout the sixteenth and seventeenth centuries

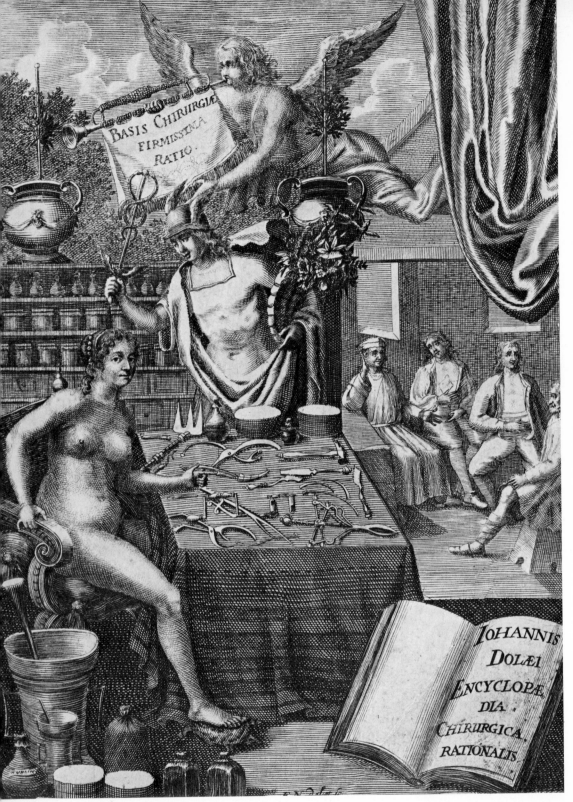

To discredit the quacks, many volumes were published basing medical practice on Reason. This title-page shows Reason, with a fine collection of surgical instruments, ready to operate on the four patients in her waiting room

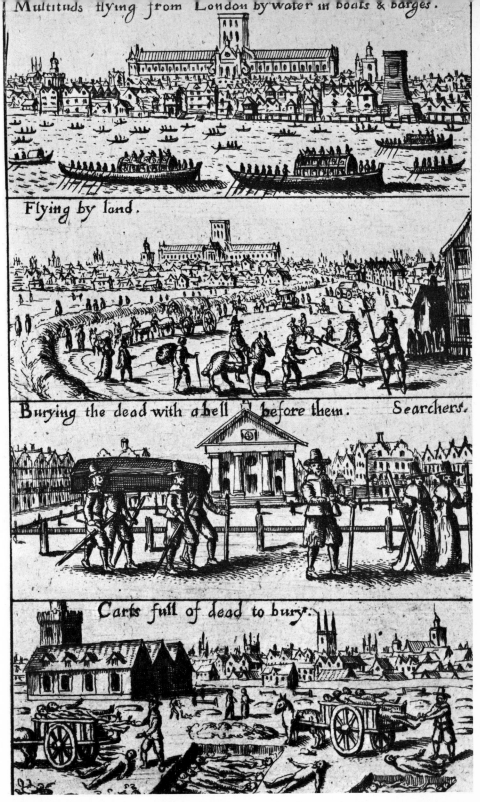

Multituds flying from London by water in boats & barges.

Flying by land.

Burying the dead with a bell before them. Searchers.

Carts full of dead to bury.

Neither Reason nor patent medicines helped against the Plague. The illustration shows scenes from the plague of 1665 in London

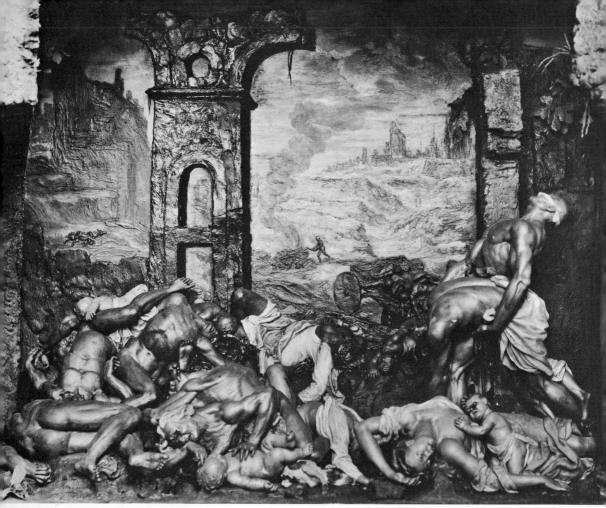

The Plague: an allegorical sculpture
in wax by Gaetano Zumbo

Two doctors dissecting the body
of a plague victim. From a treatise
on the plague published in London
in 1666

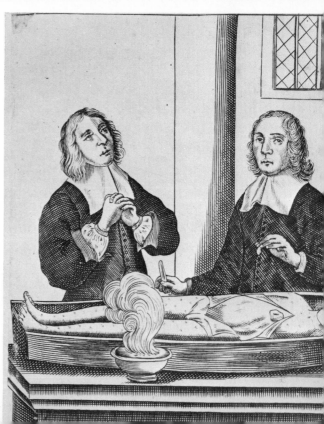

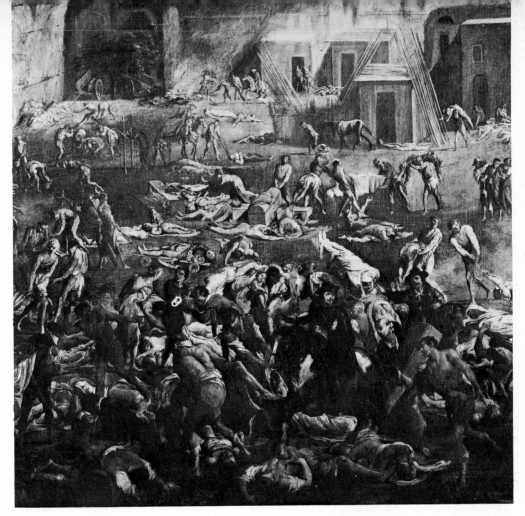

The plague of 1656 at Naples.
Detail from a painting by the
contemporary Neapolitan, Micco
Spadara

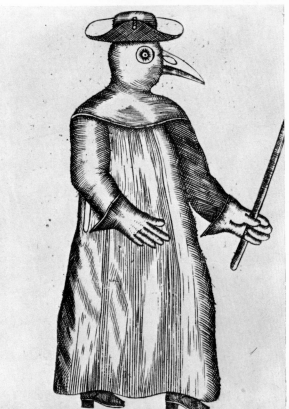

Protective clothing of the kind
worn by plague doctors during the
seventeenth century

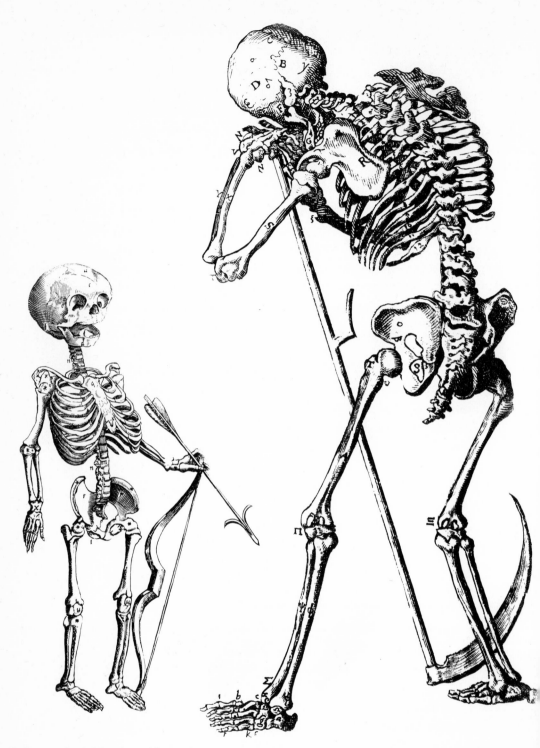

Skeletons of a child and an old man from a work on anatomy — vivid allegories of the shortness of love, and the certainty of death

How often the royal touch worked is not recorded, but it was at least as likely to succeed as the drugs of that era. And even at this late stage the distinction has to be made between belief in the occult – which was understandable, and could be therapeutically effective – and gullibility about it. Francis Bacon was a believer in astrology, and particularly in the influence of the moon; but his beliefs reflect less credulity than a genuine desire to explain the inexplicable. In general, though, the magic and the astrology were no longer, as they had been in some earlier civilisations, integral to the community's way of life. They reflected not so much active instinct as an inability to relate instinct to the new despot, intellect; they were the tribute that awareness continued to pay in order to silence the grumblings of the unconscious.

The chief advances in the period were made not in medicine, as such, but in preparing the way for a more rational approach to medicine through science. The Dutch draper Van Leeuwenhoek ground lenses to make improved microscopes, finding animalcules, far too small to be seen by the naked eye, swarming in water and in his own saliva: his discoveries, so far from bringing him before the Inquisition, were discussed and accepted at the Royal Society, founded in London in 1665 for the advancement of science – several such bodies emerged at this time: one had already been founded in Rome, and the French *Académie des Sciences* followed in 1666. All over Europe researchers began to repair the damage done by the demolition of Galen, branching out in new directions; work aptly illustrated by the celebrated drawing of Sanctorius – the inventor of the clinical thermometer – in his balance chair, in which he used to have his meals and even sleep, the better to study his metabolism, and the effect on it not only of eating and of resting, but also of emotional changes.

The researcher who made the greatest contribution was William Harvey. Harvey had qualified in Padua, where the anatomical tradition established by Vesalius still flourished; and when he was appointed physician to St Bartholomew's hospital in 1609 he was already interested less in his patients than in the workings of their bodies. The Galenic theory still held: that the human body was continually manufacturing fresh blood to replace the old stagnant blood, which was then eliminated. Harvey's researches convinced him that this was mistaken: that blood circulated. To assert this in print, though, would put him in a delicate situation. His career was going well – he won a professorship in 1615, and three years later was appointed physician to the king; he realised that to publish such revolutionary findings might jeopardise his future. For over ten years he waited, before allowing the publication of *De Motu Cordis*, generally conceded to be one of the great landmarks of medical research.

Harvey's right to be regarded as the first man to propound the theory of the circulation of the blood has been disputed. More than 3000 years earlier a Chinese emperor, Hwang Ti, had suggested that blood circulated continuously under the control of the heart. But this idea had been forgotten, or ignored – as had Servetus's. Harvey's standing in the profession made it impossible for his colleagues to ignore *De Motu Cordis*, or to submit him to the same punishment that has so often been the lot of innovators; all they could do in public was to insist that Harvey was wrong – and savagely to denigrate him in private. 'I have heard him say', John Aubrey recalled, 'that after his book on the circulation of the blood came out, he fell mightily in his practice, and that it was believed by the vulgar that he was crack-brained; and all the physicians were against his opinion, and envied him.' But Harvey was more fortunately placed than most to survive such a campaign of denigration; and in any case other researchers on the Continent, notably Marcello Malpighi, quickly confirmed and amplified his thesis. 'In about 20 or 30 years' time', Aubrey was gratified to note, 'it was received in all the universities in the world and, as Mr Hobbes says in his book *De Corpore*, he is the only man, perhaps, that ever lived to see his own doctrine established in his life time.'

Malpighi had been born in the year that *De Motu Cordis* was published; and like Harvey – and like Vesalius – he was to know success while still very young: he was still in his twenties when appointed professor of theoretical medicine at Pisa. He was also to experience the rancorous stupidity of colleagues when they found him expounding new doctrines, the legend being that they all withdrew from one of his lectures, leaving a single listener behind – the Neapolitan Giovanni Borelli, who was to share Malpighi's labours. Malpighi was the first to use the microscope for systematic anatomical research, to investigate the structure of individual organs of the body; and in the process completed Harvey's work by finding how blood flows to and from arteries to veins.

As with Harvey's work, Malpighi's was important for its impact on medical teaching and research, rather than on treatment; but at the time Harvey was serving King Charles I in the civil war, there was on the Cromwellian side a soldier, not yet a doctor, who was to revolutionise the theory of the treatment of diseases.

For a variety of reasons – the service in the Cromwellian ranks being one of them – Thomas Sydenham did not begin to devote himself seriously to medical practice until middle age: he was over forty when he qualified. He had been interested in the subject before, but had been able to regard medicine with what turned out to be valuable detachment. Spared in his youth the ruthless conditioning in pseudo-Galenism which still passed for instruction in medicine, he kept an open mind, and came to grasp the disparity between the medical teaching of his day and actual clinical experience. Although the traditional 'humors' provided him with a framework, he reconstructed the Galen edifice – converting it, as it were, into flats; he began to base his clinical practice not on a general theory of disease, but on what he saw:

After studying medicine for a few years at the University of Oxford, I returned to London and entered upon the practice of my profession. As I devoted myself with all possible zeal to the work in hand it was not long before I realised thoroughly that the best way of increasing one's knowledge of medicine is to begin applying, in actual practice, such principles as one may already have acquired; and thus I became convinced that the physician who earnestly studies, with his own eyes – and not through the medium of books – the natural phenomena of the different diseases, must necessarily excel in the art of discovering what, in any given case, are the true indications as to the remedial measures that should be employed. This was the method in which I placed my faith, being fully persuaded that if I took nature for my guide I should never stray far from the right road, even if from time to time I might find myself traversing ground that was wholly new to me.

Sydenham, in short, was a follower of Hippocrates; and it has often been said of him that he did for sixteenth-century medicine what Hippocrates had done for his time, two thousand years before. Considering what patients had to put up with in the way of treatment at that time, those who had Sydenham for their doctor could consider themselves fortunate indeed. His fundamental therapeutic belief was that the life force must be assisted, stimulated, kept in trim; he prescribed fresh air, horse-riding, and beer – in moderation: everything in moderation. His attitude was very similar to Paré's, though without the emphasis on God. He treated patients; the life force healed them.

Sydenham objected, therefore, to the prevailing doctrine of the contraries, and to polypharmacy. Where he prescribed drugs, they were 'simples'. How far the herbs he recommended were of intrinsic value cannot now accurately be estimated; but there are indications that the herbalism which flourished in Britain at this time would repay closer examination. In addition to the *materia medica* of Dioscordes and others, there was a long rural tradition of herb-prescribing for various disorders; and the two had been fused in the sixteenth century with the appearance of herbals like Culpeper's, which became a standard work. By Culpeper's time, however, herbalism had been thoroughly infiltrated with astrology and, inevitably, faith in herbs' unaided powers had diminished. Yet some of those he recommended have been used to the present day, their qualities recognised by orthodoxy – the juice of willow leaves, for example, recommended for fevers, was to acquire respectability as salicylic acid, a base for drugs used for the same purpose.

Sydenham's experience with simples and their effects, coupled with his respect for the life force, led him not merely to advocate restraint, which he found to be more effective than massive dosage, but also to propound the theory that a patient's symptoms are not the effect of his disease, but of his body's struggle to overcome the disease. This had been a commonplace among herbalists; they used to instruct patients not to be alarmed at the effect of a remedy – it was a sign that the remedy was working. Sydenham agreed. Certain diseases, he thought,

are caused by particles which are disseminated throughout the atmosphere, which possess qualities antagonistic to the humors of the body, and which – when once they gain an entrance into the system – become mingled with the blood and thus are distributed throughout the entire organism. Certain other diseases owe their origin to fermentations or putrefactions of the humors, which vary in their nature – in some cases the humors being excessive in quantity, while in others they are bad in quality; and in either event the body finds itself incapable of first assimilating them and then excreting them – a state of affairs which cannot continue beyond a certain length of time without producing further harmful effects.

What the patient regards as the symptoms of his disease, Sydenham continued, are not the work of the maleficent particle wafted in through the atmosphere, or the putrefaction of one of his humors, but the indication that his life force is doing its best to destroy, assimilate or excrete the offenders, so that they cannot establish themselves in the patient's body. What people thought of as an acute disease, therefore, should really often be considered 'a helpful effort made by nature to drive out of the body, or system, in any way possible, the morbific material'.

Sydenham found a striking example of his thesis in quinine, which began to appear in Europe early in the 1630s: the first really effective drug for a specific disorder – malaria – rather than for humoral unbalance. To Sydenham, quinine was a vindication. It cured a particular type of fever, and it did so not allopathically, by cooling down the patient, but by actually stoking up his fever – encouraging nature's fiery resistance to agents of disease. The significance of this type of treatment, though, was not to be understood until some years later, when Hahnemann explored it.

In his own day, Sydenham's writings made more impact abroad than in England, where the forceful way in which he expressed his opinions annoyed his colleagues. He was not elected to the College of Physicians; his comment 'physic is not to be learned by going to the universities; one might as well send a man to Oxford to learn shoemaking as practising physic' was hardly calculated to endear him to that university-dominated body. According to a friend – the Scots doctor Andrew Browne – Sydenham, 'who throughout his life gave the clearest proof of nobility of soul, generosity and clear-sightedness, died with accusation hanging over his head that he was "an impostor and an assassin of humanity"'. But in his lifetime he had borne slights with equanimity: having, in his own words, weighed in the balance 'whether it is better to serve men, or be praised by them' – and opted for service. Time was to avenge him, for his was to become the most respected name in the history of British medicine; and the College, much though it would have liked to, did not have the face to make his election retrospective.

Yet in the end, medical orthodoxy had the last word. Although Sydenham was canonised as 'the English Hippocrates'; his insistence on Hippocratic methods in treatment, and his criticisms of allopathy were ignored. What was remembered was the way he had described and defined individual diseases, so that henceforth they could be regarded as entities. Sydenham's importance, it has continually been emphasised, was that 'he brought doctors out of the laboratories into the sick room'. He did; but what he saw and accurately described there, was to send later generations of doctors back to their laboratories, to try to find the causes of the disease entities which he had described. In this they were later to be spectacularly successful, linking particular diseases to particular agents; and Sydenham has enjoyed much of the credit, for having pointed the way. Ironically, the way was to lead to reliance on the very kind of treatment he had set his face against: drugs destined simply to banish symptoms, often without considering whether they might be the work not of a virus or a peccant humor, but of the patient's life force.

Not long before Sydenham died, in 1689, there was a striking indication of how little his views had permeated orthodox medicine. In his *The Last Days of Charles II*, Raymond Crawfurd collected the evidence for what happened when the king fell ill:

Sixteen ounces of blood were removed from a vein in his right arm with immediate good effect. As was the approved practice at this time, the King was allowed to remain in the chair in which the convulsions seized him; his teeth were held forcibly open to prevent him biting his tongue; the regimen was, as Roger North pithily describes it, 'first to get him to wake, and then to keep him from sleeping'. Urgent messages had been dispatched to the King's numerous personal physicians, who quickly came flocking to his assistance: they were summoned regardless of distinctions of creed and politics, and they came. They ordered cupping-glasses to be applied to his shoulders forthwith, and deep scarification to be carried out, by which they succeeded in removing another eight ounces of blood. A strong antimonial emetic was administered, but as the King could be got to swallow only a small portion of it, they determined to render assurance doubly sure by a full dose of Sulphate of Zinc. Strong purgatives were given, and supplemented by a succession of clysters. The hair was shorn close and pungent blistering agents were applied all over his head; and as though this were not enough, the red-hot cautery was requisitioned as well. So severe were the convulsions that the physicians at first despaired of his life, but in some two hours consciousness was completely restored.

That was only the beginning: no less than thirteen doctors were soon in consultation, suggesting fresh remedies, until the patient died.

The New Systematists

All over Europe – with Galenism ceasing to be mandatory, with sorcery losing its hold, and with the Church's authority diminished by religious divisions – medicine was ceasing to have an accepted framework. Craving for certainty, or at least for the appearance of it, doctors began to look for a replacement. Until one was found, Galen could not be rejected; along with Hippocrates and the Arabian authorities he was still taught at medical schools, with such modifications as had become acceptable. The majority of doctors, therefore, still accepted the humoral hypothesis, and treated illness with contraries, imagining that the clinical practice followed logically from the theory. But – as had happened fifteen hundred years before, in the days of the systematists (and as was continually happening to Christian sects laying down diametrically opposed codes of conduct according to their interpretation of the Bible) the types of treatment varied according to fashion and whim; bringing theory and practice alike into the contempt which Molière expressed in *L'Amour Médecin*:

SGANAREL: Nay, gentlemen, speak one after another, pray now.

MR THOMÈS: Sir, we have reasoned upon your daughter's distemper; and in my opinion, as for my part, is that it proceeds from a great heat of blood: so I'd have you bleed her as soon as you can.

MR FONANDRÈS: And I say that her distemper is a putrefaction of humours, occasioned by too great a repletion, therefore I'd have you give her an emetic.

MR THOMÈS: I maintain that an emetic will kill her.

MR FONANDRÈS: And I, that bleeding will be the death of her.

MR THOMÈS: It belongs to you indeed to set up for a skilful man!

MR FONANDRÈS: Yes, it does belong to me; and I'll cope with you in all kinds of learning.

MR THOMÈS: Do you remember the man you killed a few days ago?

MR FONANDRÈS: Do you remember the lady you sent into the other world three days since?

MR THOMÈS: (*To Sganarel*) I have told you my opinion.

MR FONANDRÈS: (*To Sganarel*) I have told you my thoughts.

MR THOMÈS: If you don't bleed your daughter out of hand, she's a dead woman.
(*Goes out*)

MR FONANDRÈS: If you do bleed her, she'll not be alive in a quarter of an hour hence.
(*Goes out*)

Within the profession, however, the dissatisfaction with traditional theories, and the longing for a better understanding of disease and how to treat it, began in the seventeenth century to express itself in the proliferation of new systems of medicine, each with its messiah – and each with his disciples, fervently preaching ideas often very different from their master's.

The similarity of the resulting arguments to those of the earlier dogmatics, empirics and methodists is comical; and so are the various cults' inconsistencies. Outwardly the chief division was between what came to be known as the iatrochemical and iatrophysical schools. Most of the iatrochemists were vitalists – that is, they believed in the existence of a life force, along the lines of Paracelsus's archeus, as distinct from physical and chemical forces. The iatrophysicists by contrast were more materialist – more mathematically minded. But they were not consistent in their theories, still less in their practice.

The man usually regarded as the founder of the iatrochemists is Jan van Helmont of Brussels – though he might have passed on the credit to Paracelsus, whose works, even if he did not accept them in their entirety, had brought him some way along the road he was to take. His theories, like those of his master, are difficult to expound, a compound of the empirical and the mystical. The life force, he thought, directs the affairs of the human constitution. Ordinarily it preserves our equilibrium; but this can be disturbed by diseases caused either by internal disintegration or by external agents. A patient's symptoms, therefore, are ordinarily an indication that his life force is campaigning vigorously against its enemies. Like Sydenham, he felt that the campaign should be assisted, not thwarted; thus, somebody troubled by a fever should be given a fever-inducing drug. The conventional doctrine of contraries appeared to van Helmont to be a dangerous delusion; in particular, when it led to 'the blood-stained Moloch' – bleeding.

But this aspect of his teaching was soon forgotten. What was to attract disciples, and to lead to the development of a recognisable school of clinical thought, was van Helmont's belief that disease, though ordinarily due to some failure of the life force, manifests itself in a chemical change of the body's tissues, usually in a particular organ; and that treatment could also be chemical, directed to the organ concerned. To that end, van Helmont embarked on intensive research into chemistry; his discovery of carbonic acid, and his coining of the term 'gas' (in its colloquial sense of a substance having the same qualities as air) helping to make his reputation in this field. But his more philosophical theories of medicine attracted relatively little attention at the time – except from the Inquisition, which harassed him, in spite of an unblemished reputation for piety: he was on trial when he died, in 1644.

Of the iatrochemists who followed him, the best known was Franz de la Boë, or Sylvius, as he styled himself. In 1658 Sylvius was appointed to the chair of medicine at Leyden, and he proceeded to use his lectern as a pulpit from which to expound his belief in the importance of chemistry. His theories had the attraction of simplicity: particularly the use of acids to counteract any excess of alkali, and vice versa, which was ultimately to introduce bicarbonate of soda to sufferers from indigestion. But the range of iatrochemistry was inevitably restricted until its practitioners could find the actual causes, or agents, of the diseases that they were fighting against. Until then, the appropriate remedy could only be found by trial and error; and hits were infrequent.

A rival faction of iatrochemists, therefore, gained the ascendancy for a time: the vitalist or animist school of Georg Ernst Stahl, born in Germany in 1660, and the author of innumerable tendentious treatises. Stahl carried Descartes' idea of the separation of body and soul a stage further, arguing that if the soul can exist and act independently of the body, it should be capable of seeing, perhaps even of foreseeing, any threat presented by disease agents; and that it was reasonable to suppose that the soul would thereupon automatically issue instructions to the body to take the appropriate action. It followed that van Helmont had been right, up to a point; 'contraries' and other standard remedies like bleeding were to be avoided. But although Stahl was also an ardent researcher in chemistry – he was responsible for the soon-to-be-notorious phlogiston theory – he did not allow this to push him in the direction taken by van Helmont. If disease came from some breakdown in nature's signalling system, he argued, doctors should worry not about the patient's symptoms, but about how to put the system to rights.

This was all very well – but how? His contemporary William Cullen complained that the vitalist system had a baneful influence on treatment, 'as either leading physicians into, or continuing them in, a weak and feeble practice, and at the same time superseding or discouraging all the attempts of art' – the 'attempts of art' being the various drugs in the *materia medica*. And Cullen's point about the Stahlian system having a baneful effect on practice was not simply the jealousy of the practitioner of a rival school. Then, as always, the doctor who appeared to his patients to be doing little or nothing for them might well be failing them, even though at the time there was little he could do that would be clinically effective; because he was not giving them the reassurance they craved, and often got, from bleeding or from a drug.

What Cullen was saying about the iatrochemists was, roughly, what Asclepiades had said about the Hippocratic school: that any positive treatment was better than their 'meditation upon death'. It became desirable, therefore, for the iatrochemists to manoeuvre themselves back into a

105

position where they could at least appear to be giving active treatment; and the change was ingeniously, though not consciously, performed by a slight shift on the subject of the archeus, or life force. Friedrich Hoffman, a colleague of Stahl's at the university of Halle, agreed with him that the life force kept the body in that state of equilibrium which we call health. He felt, though, that this was not a negative state: the force was a 'tonus', which needed to be kept up to the mark, and although there might be occasions when illness arose out of an excess of tonus, much more commonly it was caused by a deficiency – in which case a 'tonic' was needed.

Hoffman's was only one of several variations on vitalism: another was put forward by Albrecht von Haller – the presiding genius, as he has been described, of eighteenth-century medicine: poet, novelist, bibliographer, naturalist as well as author of a full-scale work on physiology. Von Haller took up an earlier notion of the life force as operating through 'irritability' – the capacity to react to stimuli, which enables the body or its various parts to make the appropriate reaction when affected by stimuli – changes of pressure, temperature and so on: his work can be regarded as an early venture into behaviourism. But from the point of view of its effect on treatment, the system which had most importance was the one propounded by the Scot, John Brown, in his *Elementa Medicinae*, published in 1780. That Brown had originally been destined for the ministry reflected no saintliness of character; drink and debts were to land him in prison. But his *Elementa Medicinae* was one of those books which for no obvious reason capture the imagination of readers – perhaps because Brown made everything seem so simple. Life, he taught, is a state of permanent excitation, maintained by stimuli, emotional and physical: ill-health is simply a maladjustment of the stimuli, either because they are in excess (like a bellows used so fiercely that it tends to blow the fire out) or, much more commonly, they suffer from a deficiency (like a bellows used so gently that the fire dies down). Illnesses, therefore, are of two categories: sthenic, which require sedation; or asthenic, needing something to stir the life force into greater activity.

Not only are the resemblances striking between these theories and those of the systematists centuries before; so is the way in which the theories were ingeniously but arbitrarily linked to therapeutic practice. The Brunonians (as Brown's followers came to be known) claimed that the symptoms of a disorder were of little relevance except insofar as they gave an indication whether sthenia or asthenia was indicated. Treatment, therefore, was based on the answers to three questions: is the disease sthenic or asthenic? Is it general or local? And what is its degree? These questions answered, it was a matter merely of choosing from quite a small range of appropriate remedies, ranging from opium (a stimulant), to bleeding (a debilitant), with amounts regulated according to the patient's needs and condition.

But simple though this sounded, it begged the question of the patient's needs and condition. How much – of a stimulant or a debilitant – was enough? The Brunonians quickly won an unenviable reputation as believers in massive doses of drugs; so much so that one of their critics was to accuse them of causing more casualties than the Terror and the Bonapartist wars put together. There was furious controversy between the Brunonians and rival medical cults, leading to violence – the police had to be called in to put down one riot at a Continental university. And the Brunonian theory spread to America, largely through the enthusiasm of the commanding medical figure there of his time: Benjamin Rush, a friend of Franklin's and a passionate advocate of the rights of man: of colonists, of negroes, of minority religions, of the insane. He became no less involved in Brunonianism, believing that yellow fever was a sthenic condition, and treating patients with massive doses of drugs and heavy bleedings which were unlikely to improve their prospects – though, as Sigerist charitably remarked, 'in the hands of a great physician all theories achieve results'.

Where the iatrochemists tended to be vitalists, the iatrophysicists were mechanistic – or, as they would have preferred to be regarded, mathematical in their attitude. They thought of the body as a machine; and they assumed that if the machinery could be fully understood, disease would be too. In this they were in the tradition of Sanctorius; but iatrophysics did not begin to emerge as a cult until it was propounded by Descartes in his treatise on physiology, published after his death in 1662. His physiology turned out to be inaccurate, which prevented the book from sharing the reputation of his philosophical works; but his ideas about the importance of the nervous system were later to be accepted and developed along behavouristic lines.

Iatrophysics was particularly influential in Italy, where it was taken up in the seventeenth century by Borelli, at Pisa, and Giorgio Baglivi, Professor of Anatomy in Rome; but the man chiefly responsible for bringing it into the main stream of European medicine was Hermann Boerhaave. Like Brown, Boerhaave had not at first intended to take up a medical career; he was due to follow his father into the ministry until, if legend is correct, some words lightly spoken in defence of Spinoza brought him under suspicion of doctrinal deviation. It was medicine's gain: Boerhaave stands in much the same commanding position in the eighteenth century as Sydenham had in the seventeenth. Sydenham's influence, though, was relatively slight in his lifetime; Boerhaave probably had more direct effect on his contemporaries and pupils than any other doctor in history.

Inevitably, legends sprang up around him; so many students flocked in from other countries to hear him lecture, it was said, that no lecture theatre was big enough to hold them. They found him – to quote his pupil von Haller's eulogy – 'a truly divine character, in his goodness to all, in his benevolence even to the envious and to rivals. No one ever heard him say a disparaging word.' And his pupils went out from Leyden to practise, write and teach in their own countries with a fresh attitude of mind that von Haller typified.

Boerhaave regarded himself as an eclectic: he did not try to squeeze what he had extracted from the different schools of medical thought into too narrow a system. Students came to him not so much for theory, as for sound clinical sense. Patients' case histories were meticulously recorded; diagnosis followed (Boerhaave's reputation as a diagnostician stood extremely high, which meant that patients whose doctors could not find out what was the matter with them came to him from all over Europe); then prognosis, in the Hippocratic pattern; then, advice on the course of treatment.

By later generations of doctors, however, Boerhaave was chiefly to be remembered less for his eclecticism than for his reiteration of the need for a more scientific spirit in medicine – as against abstractions. 'Every vital action depends on certain bodily conditions and relations; every change in these bodily conditions and relations is necessarily followed by a corresponding change in the vital activity; medicine, therefore, must be based on physiology.' In effect, he was saying – as Sylvius had done, but without the emphasis on chemistry – that even if some failure of the life force was the cause of ill-health, the illness itself was a physical end-product; if, therefore, some way could be found to reverse the end-product, this could be effective in treating the disease – an interesting prognosis of the type of treatment that began to dominate medicine in the twentieth century.

And although Boerhaave revered Sydenham – doffing his headgear, if legend is correct, every time the great physician's name was mentioned – this did not prompt him to following Sydenham's bedside ways. Boerhaave was prepared to accept such vigorous measures as bleeding until the patient fainted, or heavy doses of drugs. For most eighteenth-century patients, in fact, it was often immaterial whether their doctor favoured the iatrophysical or iatrochemical schools: the treatment he prescribed might be little different from that which Galen had initiated centuries before.

If anything, it was harsher; because when contraries were being used to fight disease, it appeared to stand to reason that the more powerful the contrary, the more rapidly the disease would be brought under control. As a result, the methods used to shorten King Charles II's last illness became a commonplace, to the point when the heavy doses of unpleasant drugs, frequent bleeding or cupping, and the application of clysters, purges and sudorifics began to cause a revulsion. As theories increased – John Wesley, the founder of the religious Methodist sect, complained in his *Primitive Physick*, published in 1768:

simple medicines were more and more disregarded . . . in room of these, abundance of new ones were introduced, by reasoning speculative men; and those more and more difficult to be applied, as being more remote from common observation. Hence rules for the application of those, and medical books, were immensely multiplied; till at length physic became an abstruse science, quite out of reach of the ordinary man.

What was worse, Wesley went on to complain, was that doctors found that to be abstruse often raised their reputation; patients thought that what was unintelligible must be remarkable. So they began to introduce 'abundance of compound medicines, neither the names nor nature of which their own countrymen understood . . . and thus both their honour and their gain was secured, a vast majority of mankind being utterly cut off from helping either themselves or their neighbours, or daring to attempt it'. A typical example was theriac, a concoction believed to have been discovered by Mithridates the Great of Pontus as an antidote against poisons. By Galen's time theriac contained seventy-three ingredients, made up into pills the size of grapes, to be taken in quantity before and after meals: and variants were still being so extensively used in the eighteenth century that they aroused William Heberden, one of Dr Johnson's doctors, to a diatribe against it.

The post-Renaissance period, then, was not a time of therapeutic advance. Few new benefits were enjoyed by the sick; and they ceased to have many of the advantages that patients had enjoyed in older times – devoted Christian care; sanitation; hygiene; diet; rest; quiet. Doctors were held in contempt by the educated; it would be easy to compile a book of invective about them appearing in seventeenth- and eighteenth-century literature: from Dryden's

> Better to hunt in fields, for health unbought
> Then fee the doctor for a nauseous draught.

– to Molière, again:

LYSETTA: What will you do, sir, with four physicians? Is not one enough to kill any one body?

SGANAREL: Hold your tongue. Four advices are better than one.

LYSETTA: Why can't your daughter die well enough without the assistance of these gentlemen?

SGANAREL: Do the physicians kill people?

LYSETTA: Undoubtedly; and I knew a man who proved by good reasons that we should never say, such a one is dead of a fever, or a catarrh, but she is dead of four doctors and two apothecaries.

SGANAREL: Don't offend these gentlemen.

LYSETTA: Faith, sir, our cat is lately recovered of a fall she had from the top of the house into the street, and was three days without either eating or moving foot or paw; but 'tis lucky for her that there are no cat-doctors, for 'twould have been over with her, and they would not have failed purging and bleeding her.

SGANAREL: Will you hold your tongue, I say? What impertinence is this! Here they come.

LYSETTA: Take care. You are going to be greatly edified; they'll tell you in Latin that your daughter is sick.

9

THE AGE OF REDISCOVERY

Preventive Medicine

THE search for medical systems which continued to preoccupy most of the best minds in medicine in the eighteenth, as well as the seventeenth century, met with little clinical success. But although the eighteenth century was not a period when any decisive new advance was made in medicine, certain therapeutic truths known to medicine earlier, but neglected or ignored by countries which regarded themselves as civilised, were rediscovered.

The first of the rediscoveries was inoculation; and its introduction to Europe via Britain can be regarded as a curious example of what W. S. Gilbert stigmatised as the idiotic habit of some of his countrymen of admiring the customs of every country but their own. On April Fool's Day, 1717, the wife of the British Ambassador at Constantinople, Lady Mary Wortley Montagu, wrote a letter to a friend at home in which she described how:

the smallpox, so fatal and general amongst us, is here entirely harmless, by the invention of engrafting which is the term they give it. There is a set of old women, who make it their business to perform the operation, every autumn, in the month of September, when the great heat is abated. People send to one another to know if any of their family has a mind to have the smallpox; they make parties for this purpose, and when they are met (commonly fifteen or sixteen together) the old woman comes with a nut-shell of the matter of the best sort of small pox, and asks what veins you please to have opened. She immediately rips open that you offer to her, with a large needle (which gives you no more pain than a common scratch) and puts into the vein as much matter as can lie upon the head of her needle ... Every year thousands undergo this operation, and the French Ambassador says pleasantly that they take the smallpox here by way of diversion, as they take the waters in other countries. There is no example of any one that has died of it, and you may believe that I am well satisfied of the safety of this experiment, since I intend to try it on my dear little son.

The origins of smallpox are obscure, but by the seventeenth century it had become probably the most feared in Europe of all the epidemic disorders – particularly because, unlike the bubonic plague, cholera or typhus it ignored social standing in its visitations. Macaulay has an affecting passage in his *History of England* on the death of Queen Mary, the wife of William of Orange:

That disease, over which science has since achieved a succession of glorious and beneficent victories, was then the most terrible of all the ministers of death. The havoc of the plague had been far more rapid: but the plague had visited our shores only once or twice within living memory; and the small pox was always present, filling the church-yards with corpses, tormenting with constant fears all whom it had not yet stricken, leaving on those whose lives it spared the hideous traces of its power, turning the babe into a changeling at which the mother shuddered, and making the eyes and cheeks of the betrothed maiden objects of horror to the lover. Towards the end of the year 1694, this pestilence was more than usually severe. At length the infection spread to the palace, and reached the young and blooming Queen. She received the intimation of her danger with true greatness of soul. She gave orders that every lady of her bedchamber, every maid of honour, nay, every menial servant, who had not had the small pox, should instantly leave Kensington House. She locked herself up during a short time in her closet, burned some papers, arranged others, and then calmly awaited her fate.

It was calculated that half the population of Europe bore the pock-marks throughout their lives as witness of having survived it; but one out of every four who caught it died. In the New World, when it was introduced, the slaughter was much heavier, massacring the natives and making their conquest much simpler than it would otherwise have been, but also continuing to ravage the immigrants. That Lady Mary should have been prepared to try it on her son was the measure not of her devotion to the cause of medical science, but of the prevailing terror of the disease, and of her relief that some means had been found to escape from it.

It seems probable that the notion of inoculation against smallpox had reached Turkey from the Far East, where it had been used for hundreds of years. One of the Indian Vedas described the process: 'put the fluid from the pustules on to the point of a needle, and introduce it into the arm, mixing the fluid with the blood; a fever will be produced, but this illness will be very mild, and need inspire no alarm.' At some stage it had even been realised that the risk from the inoculation was diminished if the fluid from the

Opposite: The Surgeon (detail) by David Ryckaert (1612–61)

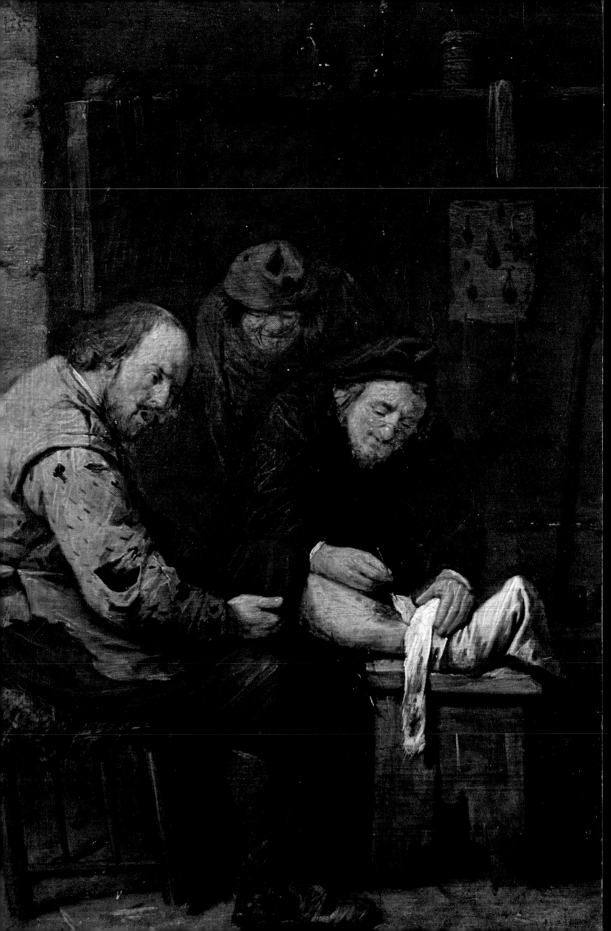

pustules was made less virulent; and various ingenious means of attenuating it had been devised. Some tribes ground up smallpox scabs in water, leaving them a few days before use; in China, ground-up scabs were blown down the nose.

Paracelsus appears to have encountered inoculation on his travels: according to his biographer John Hargrave, he used it against the plague,

he took a specimen of the patient's excreta. Then, taking a needle, he would lift upon its point the smallest speck of that infected excretal matter. This speck, so minute as to puzzle the eye to see it, he now placed in a small pellet made of bread-sop, and this he rolled into a ball or pill. Finally he administered the bread pill to the patient, making sure it was swallowed. Thus, plague cured plague; the disease was the cure, when properly prepared and reduced to an infinitesimal dose.

But this, Hargrave noted, was not quite the same principle: what Paracelsus was trying to do was less to isolate the germ or spirit of the plague, than to administer a dose of the particular plague spirit of the patient – with a view to the body's own alchemy, or archeus, working. It took the enthusiasm and social standing of Lady Mary to put across the method; she made it her business to propagate the faith, with such success that the royal children were soon inoculated (though the king insisted that it should be tried out on six condemned men in Newgate first, as a precaution).

Inoculation, though, had the defect that it was not entirely trustworthy: sometimes patients got a real, rather than a prophylactic dose. Again, it was folk medicine which gave a clue how the risk could be reduced without significant loss of protection. The discovery forms one of the most familiar stories in medical hagiology. An English country doctor, Edward Jenner happened to hear a farm girl boasting that she couldn't get smallpox because she had had cowpox; the remark stuck in his mind, nagging at him to find a way to rid humanity of that terrible scourge; and eventually he took pus from a girl infected with cowpox, transferred it to two local boys, injected them a few days later with smallpox germs – and, when they were none the worse, prepared to claim a place among the heroes of medicine.

As usual, the medical establishment was contemptuous. Jenner's account of his 'vaccination' was rejected by the Royal Society – not without reason, for it was an amateurish effort. When in 1798 he published it himself, in a short work entitled *An Inquiry into the Causes and Effects of the Variolae Vaccine*, it was received with indifference. Again, the initial enthusiasm came from abroad. In 1799 the Austrian sanitary authorities, attracted to the idea, began their own experiments, and by the winter of 1801 they had proved successful. Only on the backwash of this Continental fame did Jenner begin to acquire a reputation in his own country; in 1802 Parliament voted Jenner £10,000, and a few years later, doubled that sum in a second grant.

But after the initial enthusiasm – reflected in George Washington's order that all recruits to the United States army should receive it – vaccination began to accumulate critics. Its value and its safety were called in question, and the idea of immunising people to a disease by giving them a small attenuated dose of the virus, to give mild symptoms but also protect the constitution against later attacks, was for a time abandoned.

The second of the preventive medicine rediscoveries of this period concerned the necessity of a balanced diet. As civilisation developed, men and women not only lost their primitive instinct for eating the kind of food they needed to maintain health; they also began to live in conditions where it was unlikely their diet would be balanced. Town life was bad enough; much worse were the conditions in which sailors were forced to live. This had not mattered so much while voyages were made for the most part within sight of land, with frequent visits ashore to obtain fresh water and replenish stores; but when the crossing of the Atlantic and the Pacific began, crews were frequently forced back on heavily salted meat and hard biscuit, which deprived them of vitamins essential to health, and sometimes to life.

Far more sea battles and campaigns were lost through failure to prevent disease and death among sailors, than by inadequate armament or sail, or indifferent tactics. The records from Elizabethan times reflect a formidable mortality. Scurvy. Admiral Hawkins claimed, cost him 10,000 men during his career; and there is no reason to believe that he was outstandingly unlucky. From simple self-interest, it might be expected, the Admirality and other parties would have encouraged investigation, and experimented with possible remedies, rather than allow such a chronic (and often exceedingly dangerous) threat to their manpower to remain. Yet it was not until James Lind, a physician in a Portsmouth naval hospital, became interested in the subject in the middle of the eighteenth century that any serious investigation into the subject was undertaken. Lind's findings, published in 1757 in his

Essay on the most effectual means of preserving the health of Seamen, showed that scurvy was the result of wretched living conditions and inadequate diet; and he made one of the simplest but one of the most celebrated of therapeutic suggestions: that a ration of fresh fruit should be supplied to prevent it. It was too simple; although the proposition was successfully tested by Captain Cook – whose ship was scurvy-free throughout its voyage of well over three years in the South Seas, because he took the precaution of providing a ration of lemon juice for his men – the Admiralty remained unimpressed.

'Some persons', as Lind perceptively complained, 'cannot be brought to believe that a disease so fatal and so dreadful can be cured or prevented by such easy means. They would have more faith in an elaborate composition dignified with the title of "an antiscorbutic golden elixir" or the like.' It would be interesting to know what would have happened had Lind patented his 'elixir', and offered it to the Admiralty as a secret formula; the deal might have been profitable. But years passed before the Admiralty could be persuaded to make the experiment with anything so simple as lemon juice. It was eventually supplied to a naval squadron in the year of Lind's death, 1794; and the results of the test fully vindicated his thesis. But another ten years went by before it became standard daily issue in the navy.

For armies, at this time, fevers of various descriptions, commonly culminating in typhus, remained the main hazard; and a contemporary of Lind's, Sir John Pringle, appears to have been the first to investigate whether simple preventive measures might prove effective. While Physician-General to the forces in the campaigns of the 1740s, he noticed that epidemic fevers were rare when the soldiers were in open camps; they must, he decided, be the result of the overcrowding, the inadequate ventilation and the poor sanitary conditions of ordinary army living quarters – as well as of hospitals and jails. So he advocated smaller and better-maintained billets, hospitals and jails, and frequent changes of quarters when in the field.

Ironically, Pringle chose as a good illustration of his theme, the conditions prevailing on the island of Walcheren, off the Dutch coast, where the camp confines and dampness were well calculated, he thought, to encourage the spread of epidemic disease. Although his book had been widely read, not merely in England but in translation in many European countries, it had not apparently, been brought to the attention of the British military authorities; or perhaps they had thought Pringle's remedies, like Lind's, were too simple.

In 1809 they sent an expedition to Walcheren. It met the conditions Pringle had forecast over half a century before, with the consequences he had predicted. Within a few weeks, the local endemic fever, supplemented by typhus, had all but annihilated the expeditionary force of 40,000, leaving about one man in ten capable of bearing arms, and necessitating a humiliating evacuation of the island.

Mental Illness

The eighteenth century also saw the beginnings of a revival of Hippocrates' enlightened attitude to mental disorders. The days of the widespread epidemics of mass hysteria were past: witches were ceasing to arouse alarm, and so were witch-hunters. Belief in diabolic possession was also dwindling. It was still not uncommon, though, for artificially induced hysteria to appear in religious communities – and even to be exploited as a technique of conversion; notably, as William Sargant showed in his *Battle for the Mind*, by John Wesley, the founder of the religious sect of Methodists. The 'Quakers', 'Shakers', 'Rollers' and other groups behaved not very differently from medieval communities afflicted by the dancing mania, or nuns possessed by devils. Wesley's journal is full of examples:

While I was speaking one before me dropped down as dead, and presently a second and a third. Five others sunk down in half an hour, most of whom were in violent agonies. The 'pains of hell came about them, the snares of death overtook them'. In their trouble we called upon the Lord, and He gave us an answer of peace. One indeed continued an hour in strong pain, and one or two more for three days; but the rest were greatly comforted in that hour, and went away rejoicing and praising God.

The fact that such manifestations were premeditated – spontaneous hysteria of the kind common in earlier centuries having become infrequent – did not work out to the benefit of the mentally ill. The pleas of Paracelsus, Vives and Weyer had been forgotten; it was no longer assumed that lunatics were possessed by the devil, or, as their name implied, in thrall to some cosmic catastrophe, but in the absence of any satisfactory explanation for their irrationality they were cruelly treated.

How cruelly can be gauged from one of the earliest pleas for a new attitude to insanity for social as distinct from psychiatric reasons. It was advanced by

Daniel Defoe, years before he obtained notoriety as a journalist, and then fame as an author. As well as advocating that the mentally defective and the insane should be separated, he warned that unscrupulous people were putting away relations, particularly wives they wanted to get rid of, in institutions.

If they are not mad when they go into these cursed houses, they are soon made so by the barbarous usage they there suffer . . . is it not enough to be suddenly clapped up, stripped, whipped, ill-fed and worse used? To have no reason assigned for such treatment, no crime alleged, no accusers to confront? And, what is worse, no soul to appeal to but merciless creatures, who answer to laughter, surliness, contradiction, and too often stripes?

It should be made a crime, Defoe urged, to confine anybody in a madhouse without due authority; and for the really insane, licensed institutions should be set up, subject to proper visitation and inspection.

Defoe's idea was not to reach the statute book until 1774: and in the meantime the insane continued to be badly treated – with the additional humiliation that they came to be looked on as comic. People went to watch lunatics much as they might now go to the monkey-house at the zoo, for a good laugh. The member of a well-to-do family who began to suffer from a mental disorder would ordinarily be cared for in a private institution; but the great majority, lacking means, were herded together in brutish conditions with no heat – frostbite was commonly reported – no clothes (if they were torn off, or if they wore out, no replacement was available) poor lighting and inadequate ventilation. Inmates were chained to the walls, and gagged if they had been violent or obstreperous. Nothing that can reasonably be described as treatment was given – though ducking in cold water had its advocates as a way to bring unruly patients to their senses; or they would be bled to the point of physical exhaustion. Where they continued refractory their actions were considered not as an indication that their disorder required different treatment, but as a crime deserving of punishment.

As has so often happened in the history of medicine, two men in two different countries who were revolted by the treatment of the insane were moved to action at the same time. In England, William Tuke founded the York Retreat for the mentally disordered, where they found themselves in a hospital rather than in prison conditions. This was in 1792; and the following year in Paris, Philippe Pinel acquired more durable fame by striking the fetters off some of the inmates of the Bicêtre in Paris. Pinel had become interested in the insane because of the fate of a friend who had gone mad, and been locked up; he had escaped from the institution and fled to a forest, where his skeleton was found later – the presumption being that he had been devoured by wolves. Convinced that deprivation of liberty, and particularly of movement, was actually a cause of madness, Pinel decided to make the experiment of freeing selected prisoners – for prisoners in effect they were – and observing the consequences. His opportunity came when he was appointed to the Bicêtre. It was in 1793, a year which made the experiment doubly dangerous, for he had first to obtain the permission of Couthon, Robespierre's lieutenant, himself a paranoiac, who suspected that aristocrats and enemies of the people were being hidden among the insane. Pinel risked his life, therefore, both from the men he released from the chains, and from the guillotine if the public were put in danger. But the liberation passed off uneventfully. One man ran away, but was soon brought back; and Pinel himself, though at times his life was in danger, survived not only through the Terror, but through all the political upheavals that followed, working on until 1826.

Pinel's philosophy was simple. As he told Couthon, 'the mentally ill are intractable only because they are deprived of fresh air and liberty'. He was a humane man, but his treatment was based less on humane than on rational considerations: he thought that crowding madmen together in unspeakable conditions was inefficient because it made them worse. He had no therapeutic notions other than treating the insane as patients, not as criminals; far from being guilty, and deserving of punishment, they were 'sick people whose miserable state deserves all the consideration that is due to suffering humanity'. His aim was simply to try to build up patients' confidence by taking them seriously, and trying to understand their problems.

Pinel, in short, has strong claims to be the founder of what was later to become known as the Open Door school of psychiatry; and he did it without therapeutic aids, tranquillisers or electric shocks. In other ways, too, he anticipated modern developments; in the care with which he kept records and case histories, and in his belief in the importance of efficient hospital administration. But the defect of his system was that it required a man of his interest and his integrity to make it work. He could handle the insane because they responded to him; they felt he was on their side, and appreciated what he was trying to do for them. Other men in charge of mental hospitals might seek to establish the same regime, only to find that individual inmates were abusing their privileges, by trying to escape or making scenes. The easy reply was to withhold privileges, as a punishment; but this aroused resentment, and before very long the doors would have to be shut again, and locked. The straitjackets and the padded cells would then come back into use, and the hospital revert to its former custodial function. A new administrator never found any difficulty in justifying such actions. He could argue that his first responsibility was for the safety of his charges, and of the public; and the public would be on his side – usually the relatives, too, who were often glad to be rid of a family nuisance. As a result, though a few individual psychiatrists continued to use humane methods with the same success as Pinel, the Open Door system did not fully establish itself until the discovery of tranquillisers; they were to make it possible to create artificially the conditions that Pinel had obtained by the force of his personality.

Mesmerism

Yet another revival of an old therapeutic idea during the eighteenth century was what can loosely be called occultism, with particular emphasis on the importance of the cosmos in relation to human health.

At the time this was widely regarded as quackery: and indeed it was often difficult to differentiate the genuine from the spurious. The eighteenth century is commonly regarded as the golden age of quackery, and with some reason. The most successful, reckoned in terms of gulling the authorities, was probably Joanna Stephens, who in the 1730s claimed that she had a cure for gallstones, which she was prepared to disclose for £5,000. When private subscriptions failed to raise that sum, the British Parliament appointed a commission, including some fashionable doctors of the day, who inquired into her cures and 'found themselves convinced by experiment of their utility and efficiency'. The £5,000 was paid over, and the inventor disclosed her prescriptions, made of such ingredients as crushed snails, powdered eggshells, burned hips and haws, soap and honey. Benjamin Franklin, then in London, was sceptical, but he appears to have been an exception – and perhaps the mixture was often effective, through suggestion.

This was even more true of one of the most celebrated nostrums in history:

the 'Celestial Bed'. It was an invention of the Scot, James Graham, whom the historian of quackery, Eric Jameson, regarded as probably the most striking representative of the quack species. In 1780 Graham opened a Temple of Health in an elegant London house on the Aesculapian design, with scantily dressed and nubile vestal virgins, or goddesses – one of them, it was later alleged, being the future Lady Hamilton, Horatio Nelson's mistress – to look after patients. The showpiece of the establishment was the Bed, advertised as being

12 feet long by 9 feet wide, supported by 40 pillars of brilliant glass of the most exquisite workmanship, in richly variegated colours. The super celestial dome of the bed, which contains the odoriferous, balmy and ethereal spices, odours and essences, which is the grand reservoir of those reviving invigorating influences which are exhaled by the breath of the music and the exhilarating force of electrical fire, is covered on the other side with brilliant panes of looking glass.

The therapeutic force was provided by fifteen hundredweight of magnets; the objective, apart from ministering to the general health of those who used it, being to assist husbands and wives to a 'genial and happy issue': conception.

The idea that magnetism could be exploited in treatment was an ancient one: Paracelsus had been attracted to it, and during the seventeenth century a number of variations on it had emerged, the best known being the method adopted by the Irish healer Valentine Greatraks, whose successes much impressed his fellow countryman Robert Boyle and other members of the Royal Society. Greatraks used the technique to cure patients that is used to magnetise an iron bar, gently stroking the afflicted part of the body. According to an eyewitness:

I had the honour to be present at the experiment made by the Right Honourable the Lord Viscount Falconbridge, upon John Jacomb of George-Alley in Southwark, whose exquisite and continual pains, by the gentle touch and easy friction of Mr Greatraks' hand, were allured out of his arm and shoulder to the extreme joints and ends of his fingers, which became thereby (as the man affirmed) devoid of sense, benumbed and dead. Whereupon his Lordship thrust a pin of about an inch long almost to the head, into one of his fingers, his eyes first close covered, without the least sign of the man's perception, or any blood appearing when the pin was pulled out. He then thrust it into another finger, as deep as the first, and asked the man if he felt nothing; who answered that he could not tell, but after a little pause, said he thought he did. Whereat my Lord admiring, pulled it out again, and Mr

The Eighteenth Century

The Dentist by Francesco Maggiotto. Dentists were not yet accepted into the medical
profession, and travelled about the country like the quacks

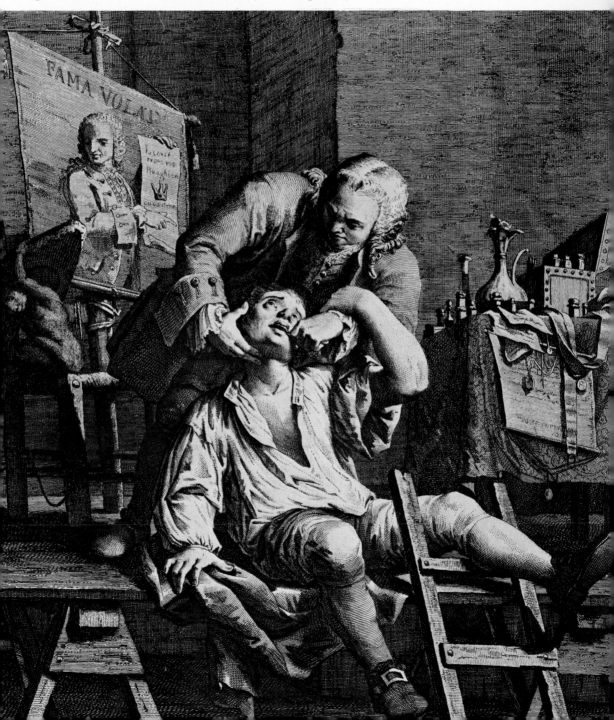

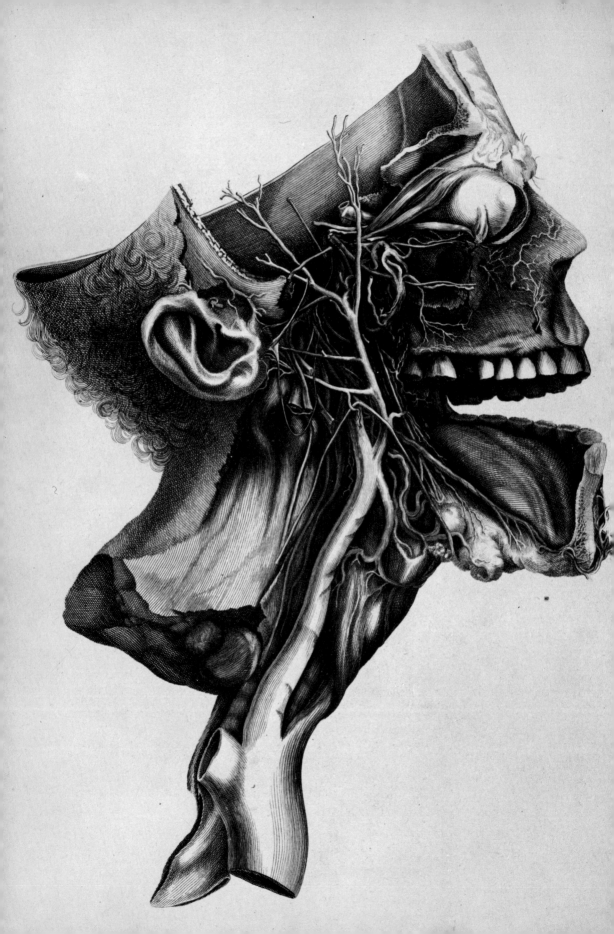

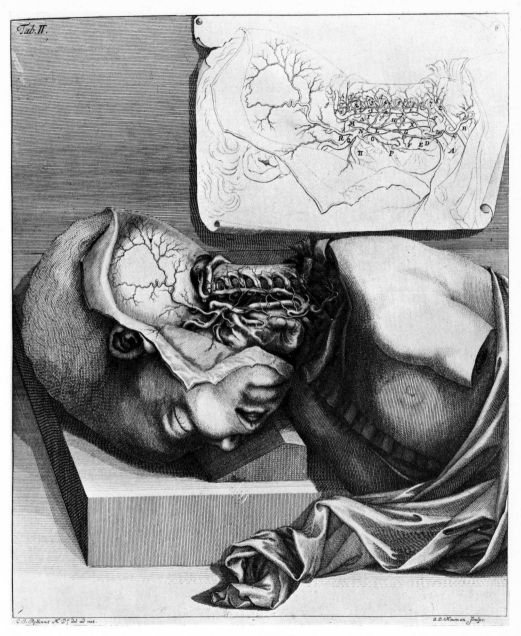

Two plates from the *Icones Anatomicae* (1743–56) of Albrecht von Haller, 'presiding genius of eighteenth-century medicine'

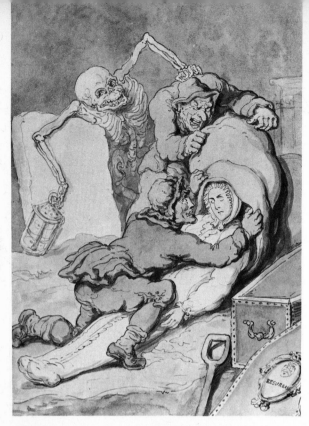

Resurrectionists by Rowlandson, stealing bodies from graveyards to be sold to the anatomy schools

Anatomy school in Great Windmill Street, London, run by the celebrated surgeon William Hunter

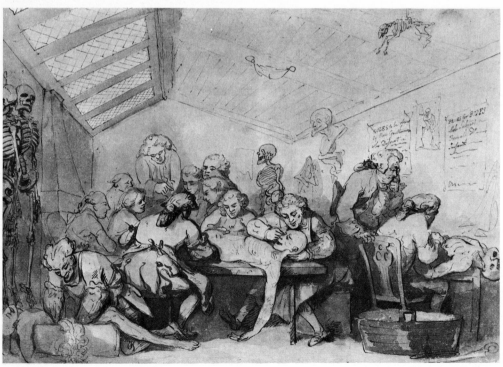

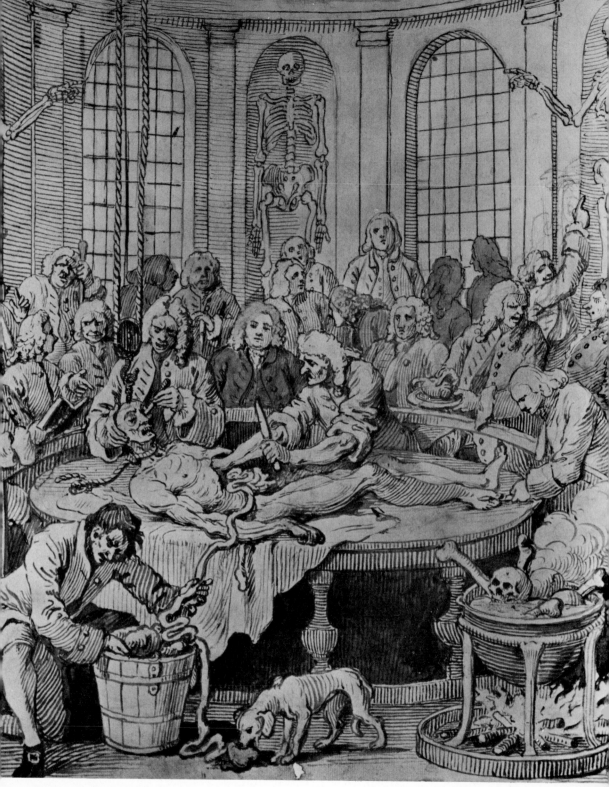

The Reward of Cruelty by Hogarth, viciously caricaturing the anatomy lessons in medical schools

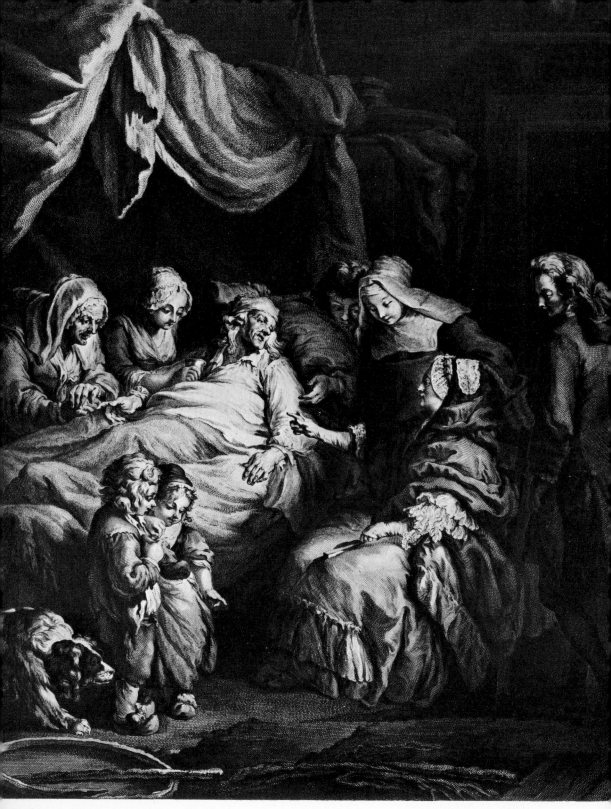

La Dame de Charité by Charles Eisen. The eighteenth century saw improvements in the treatment of the poor, and in Paris many ladies of the court devoted time to visiting the sick

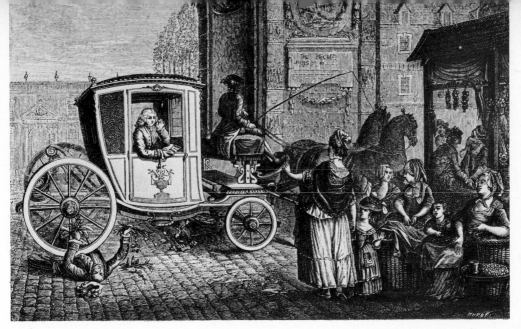

The fashionable doctor Tronchin, here seen symbolically crushing his herbalist rivals. He arrived in Paris from Geneva in 1766, and devoted two hours each day to free consultations for the poor, paying himself for their medicines

The Doctor of the Mountains in his Rustic Pharmacy (1774). The Swiss peasant Michel Schupper gained a great reputation throughout Europe for his herbal remedies

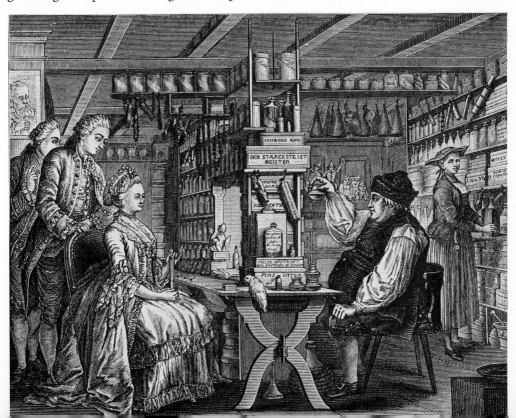

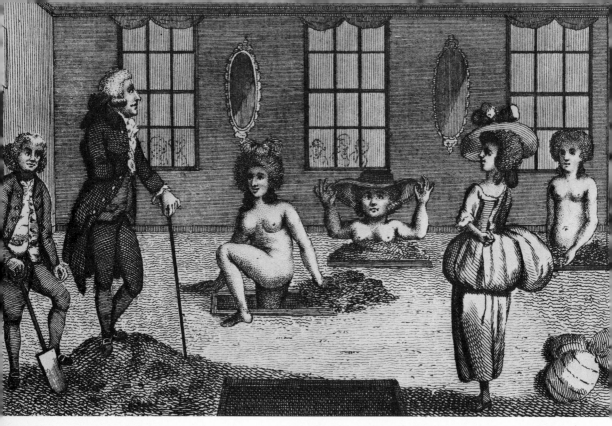

The mud baths of Dr James
Graham, inventor of the Celestial
Bed, patronized by many ladies
of fashion

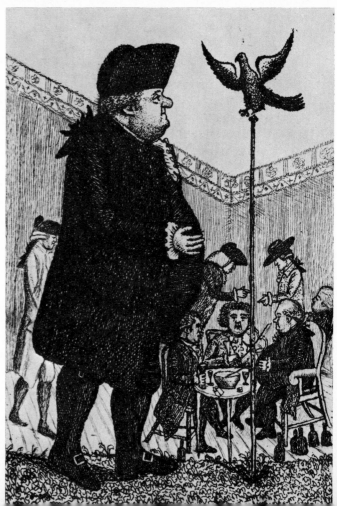

Caricature by Kay of John Brown,
founder of the Brunonians, in the
company of Graham and other
medical eccentrics

Greatraks slightly stroked the man's fingers twice or thrice, who continued blind-folded; afterwards the pin's point only touching one of his finger's ends, he smartly cried out, 'Oh, you prick me!' and blood immediately issued out of those places into which the pin had been thrust. The man professed himself freed of all pain, and may be presumed to have continued so, for he was bidden by Mr Greatraks to come again if he felt the least grudging, with promise of easy access to him, and assurance of help and ease; but hath never appeared since.

The idea that pain could be stroked out of the body continued to attract healers in the eighteenth century; some of them, like the Swiss Father Gassner, making an international reputation. And it was watching Fr Gassner that gave Franz Mesmer, born in Saxony in 1733, the idea that the power did not lie in the individual; that he was simply the medium through which the healing force was transmitted from the cosmos. It was indeed magnetism, Mesmer decided, but of an animal, not mineral, nature – though it had affinities with the mineral variety; it could also be stored in iron bars.

This was Mesmer's rationalisation; and he set out to prove that he was right. An early case established his reputation. He was fortunate in that he was of good social standing in Vienna – Mozart was a close friend; and a girl was brought to him as a patient who had attracted the sympathy and assist-ance of the Court – Maria Paradis, a skilled musician who had gone blind in infancy from paralysis of the optic nerve. Several famous surgeons had tried to cure her without success. Mesmer, taking the girl into his own house, succeeded.

The story of her recovery of her sight is full of touching episodes: such as the occasion when, on first seeing a dog, she remarked that its features were more agreeable to her than those of men. But as her eyesight returned, her parents grew worried. If she recovered altogether, she might lose the pension that the Empress had bestowed on her. The local doctors, too, resentful at Mesmer's success, sedulously spread scandals about him, suggesting that the girl had not really recovered her sight at all – a claim they were later given the chance to justify, because when she was taken against her will from Mesmer's household, she lost it again. Mesmer, outraged, decided to leave Austria; and he moved to France.

He quickly found Parisians more susceptible. The technique he evolved was to get a group of people holding or touching hands – like a spiritualist séance – round a kind of bath in which he had placed magnetised iron rods and other impedimenta; he would then appear and go through a ritual of motions designed to restore their health through the flow of animal magnetism. Some patients would go into a trance state of an active nature, with violent convulsions; others became mediums, with strange voices speaking through them, as if they had been occupied by a different personality. Others went into comas. Whatever their reaction, many felt decidedly the better for the experience.

The effect on Paris society was prodigious; overnight, to have attended Mesmer's sessions became a fashionable 'must'. So spectacular was his success that the Paris *Académie des Sciences*, which ordinarily would hardly have bothered with such matters, felt compelled to investigate mesmerism. The committee was distinguished, including Pinel, Benjamin Franklin (then US ambassador); Bailly – later unlucky enough to become mayor of Paris in 1791, an involvement in politics that was to cost him his life in the Terror; Lavoisier, and Dr Guillotin, who had invented his machine to humanise execution, and on which both Bailly and Lavoisier were to perish. They reported in 1784:

The commissioners, having convinced themselves that the animal magnetism is capable of being perceived by none of our senses, and had no action either upon themselves or upon the subjects of their several experiments; being assured that the touches and compressions employed in its application have rarely occasioned favorable changes in the animal economy, and that the impressions thus made are always hurtful to the imagination; in fine, having demonstrated by decisive experiments, that the imagination without the magnetism produces convulsions, and that the magnetism without the imagination produces nothing; they have concluded with a unanimous voice respecting the existence and the utility of the magnetism that the fluid having no existence can consequently have no use; that the violent symptoms observed in the public process are to be ascribed to the imagination called into action, and to that propensity to mechanical imitation, which leads us in spite of ourselves to the repetition of what strikes our senses.

The investigators had hit on a truth far more profound than they realised. Mesmer's theory of animal magnetism had been an attempt to explain phenomena he did not understand, but even if the theory turned out to be nonsensical, the phenomena remained to be accounted for. The investigators attributed them to imagination, and left it at that, as if it were of no significance. But by demonstrating the remarkable power of the imagination over the body in certain trance states, Mesmer had rediscovered the powers of the medicine man – an event destined to be of far-reaching significance.

Mesmer was no fraud. 'I am accused', he complained, 'of being a common cheat, and those who believe me are taunted with being fools. Such is apt to be the fate of new truths.' The elaborate hocus-pocus was part of his design: 'an excellent psychologist' Stefan Zweig described him, who 'knew that faith healing needs a certain amount of ceremonial, or magical or religious ritual, if the best results are to be achieved; he therefore surrounded himself with an atmosphere of magic'. And there was nothing disreputable about doing so. Mesmer was convinced that his animal magnetism was the clue to the mystery that had attracted magicians, sorcerers, religious mystics and philosophers; it came as no surprise to him that people reacted to his methods as they had traditionally reacted, in the days when strange contortions or anguished demonic voices had been a commonplace of healing.

What Mesmer did not realise, and it is hard to blame him, was that he was dabbling in psychological forces at once more complex and more simple than could be accounted for by animal magnetism. He did not know how effective suggestion can be, therapeutically – even when induced without the assistance of trance states; in trances its effect is simply heightened. But the 'mesmerism' of the kind Svengali used on Trilby – designed to develop latent powers or abilities (or to lead) by suggestion – was unknown to Mesmer himself. He assumed that the force was animal magnetism, flowing from the cosmos, and that it did not require any instructions from him to do its work; all he had to do was act as Master of Ceremonies, organising the séance so that the force could flow unimpeded. No doubt many of his patients went into what would now be regarded as hypnotic trances, but these were not exploited directly; Mesmer's therapeutic techniques were closer to those used by Jesus and other spiritual healers, than to hypnotherapy.

But the investigators' belief that the séances had no therapeutic effect, other than that provided by patients' imagination, was mistaken. The convulsive seizures were in the clinical line that stretches from Voodoo dances through the Tarantella to electric shock treatment: like Wesley's meetings, they provided an induced fit, of a kind which often gives the patient at least a temporary feeling of well-being. The committee may have been right in its fear that the convulsions could do harm; particularly if indiscriminately induced by doctors or quacks cashing in on the mesmerism craze. But the final justification of mesmerism, ironically, lay in the very feature that the committee had noted, and used as a crushing dismissal. It *was* the imagination of the patients, in their trance state, that counted: and Mesmer, though he did not understand the full significance of his own discovery, can hardly be denied the credit for it.

Homeopathy

Yet another eighteenth-century revival, and one that for a time had a considerable impact on medicine, was the theory of 'likes cure likes', advanced by Samuel Hahnemann. Born in Saxony in 1755, Hahnemann was an orthodox practitioner who became revolted by what appeared to him to be the inefficiency (as well as the cruelty) of allopathic treatment; and the realisation why it should so often fail came when he observed that the symptoms from a dose of quinine on a healthy body were much the same as those associated with the disease quinine was used to cure: malaria. Likes cure likes, he recalled, was to be found in Hippocrates, and in other ancient medical writings. It had appealed to Paracelsus, and it was a logical deduction from the teachings of Sydenham. If, as Sydenham had insisted, the symptoms of disease represent the efforts of the life force to throw off a morbific tendency, then quinine should be helping the life force.

In contradistinction to the prevalent allopathic theory, Hahnemann described his method as homeopathic. But he went further. In 'proving' his drugs – testing them to find out which had affinities to particular diseases – he found that the results obtained were better not merely from small doses, but from doses that were infinitesimal; diluted – or, as he thought of it, charged with potency – to the nth degree. In this he was a vitalist; he could have argued, had he thought in such terms, that it was not the mass of a substance but the energy residing in it that has curative properties.

This idea of the potency of microdoses, however, made him enemies – the chemists in particular foresaw the ruin of their trade if homeopathy should spread; and Brunonians and others who had impressed on their patients that massive doses of drugs were necessary naturally resented the implication that they were wrong. Hahnemann and his followers were bitterly assailed. Yet the movement rapidly spread: to France, where eventually Hahnemann himself went to live; to England, where it picked up socially elevated patients, and was able to survive the attacks of orthodoxy; and to the United States. The homeopathic practitioners took care not to give their enemies unnecessary opportunities to discredit them; they either qualified as doctors through recognised schools, or set up schools of their own with high standards. Their hospitals were also successful; both in London and Vienna, the mortality rate during epidemics was found to be decidedly lower in them than in orthodox institutions. By the second half of the nineteenth century homeopathy had acquired what appeared to be a secure position in medicine.

Homeopathy could also lay some claim to the paternity of immunisation, when it was revived as a therapeutic procedure in the nineteenth century. By coincidence, Hahnemann's introductory manifesto was published in the same year that Jenner implanted cowpox in the country lad, to see if it gave him immunity to smallpox – a striking example of likes curing likes. And although orthodoxy has been reluctant to give any credit for Hahnemann, it is significant that von Behring, the man who was to demonstrate that immunisation was a practical therapeutic procedure, had no doubt that he deserved it.

In spite of all scientific speculations and experiments regarding smallpox vaccination, Jenner's discovery remained an erratic block in medicine, till the bio-chemically thinking Pasteur, devoid of all medical class-room knowledge, traced the origin of this therapeutic block to a principle which cannot better be characterised than by Hahnemann's word: Homeopathic. Indeed, what else causes the epidemiological immunity in sheep, vaccinated against anthrax, than the influence previously exerted by a virus, similar in character to that fatal anthrax virus? And by what technical term could we more appropriately speak of this influence, exerted by a SIMILAR virus, than by Hahnemann's word 'Homeopathy'? I am touching here upon a subject anathematised till very recently by medical pedantry: but if I am to present these problems in historical illumination, dogmatic imprecations must not deter me.

Diagnosis

There was also, in the second half of the eighteenth century, a revival of interest in diagnosis. In spite of Sydenham's efforts, little advance had been made in it since Roman times; except perhaps uroscopy, which flourished during the Renaissance – so much so that the symbol of the physician became the carafe in which his patients' urine could be inspected. This technique has been dismissed by later commentators as 'clap-trap charlatanry' (to quote

Albert Buck; and doubtless it was often used simply as a device to impress patients; but there is no reason why doctors should not have found urine an aid to diagnosis. Uroscopy, however, went out of fashion; and there was little the doctor could do to fathom what was going on inside his patients' bodies until Leopold Auenbrugger of Vienna devised another method: percussion, described in his *Inventum Novum ex percussione thoracis humani*, published in 1761. His theory was that if the doctor rapped his patients' thorax, he could tell what was the matter by differentiating the sounds. For example

The duller the sound, and the more nearly approaching that of a fleshy limb stricken, the more severe is the disease.

The want of the natural sound behind, indicates more danger than it does on the anterior and superior part of the chest.

The total destitution of sound over one whole side, is generally a fatal sign.

Auenbrugger was under no illusions about the chances of percussion finding favour with his colleagues. 'In making public my discoveries,' he wrote, 'I have not been unconscious of the dangers I must encounter, since it has always been the fate of those who have illustrated or improved the arts and sciences by their discoveries to be beset by envy, malice, hatred, destruction and calumny.' For once this forecast was not justified – though Auenbrugger might have preferred that it had been, rather than accept the fate his book suffered. It was not denounced, it was simply ignored, until taken up by Corvisart, Napoleon's most trusted doctor, who revived the method shortly after the turn of the century.

The man who really popularised listening-in as a diagnostic aid, though, was a pupil of Corvisart's, Rene Laennec, whose life story has been described as 'one of the most touching and most heroic in the whole history of science': a long struggle with poverty and disease. To percussion, Laennec added the art of auscultation: he listened to the sounds that can be heard from various organs, usually the heart and the lungs, and diagnosed therefrom. And, seeking a way to improve his technique, he had the idea which was to provide physicians with the clinical symbol they had lacked since uroscopy went out of fashion: the stethoscope.

Laennec himself described how he got the idea in 1816, when treating a girl with heart trouble.

Owing to her stoutness little information could be gathered by application of the hand and percussion. The patient's age and sex did not permit me to resort to the kind of examination I have just described (ear to chest). I recalled a well-known acoustic phenomenon; namely, if you place your ear against one end of a wooden beam, the scratch of a pin at the other extremity is most distinctly audible ... Taking a sheaf of paper I rolled it into a very tight roll, one end of which I placed over the heart, whilst I placed my ear to the other. I was both surprised and gratified at being able to hear the beating of the heart with much greater clarity and distinctness than I had ever done before by direct application of my ear.

Up to that time, Osler commented, the clinical recognition of diseases had made very little real progress; the stethoscope enabled that progress to begin, and Laennec's work is 'in the category of the eight or ten greatest contributions to the science of medicine'. So it was to prove, but not till long after Laennec's death – of TB, ironically: the disease his stethoscope was to be so valuable in diagnosing. It took time to break down the prejudice of the profession against the new gadget. When John Elliotson introduced it to England, one of his fellow members of the College of Physicians jeered at it: 'Ah, do you use that hocus-pocus?' Elliotson insisted he found it extremely useful; he was told, 'You will learn nothing by it and, if you do, you cannot treat disease the better.' Elliotson's critic was wrong about there being nothing to learn from auscultation: for purposes of diagnosis and prognosis it was invaluable. But he was largely right that it could do little to improve the treatment of disease, which had to await better knowledge of disease processes.

A few years later, a more unusual method of detecting what was going on inside a patient was employed by a US army surgeon, William Beaumont, called in to treat a trapper who had been accidentally shot in the stomach at close range. The wound healed, leaving a small orifice through which Beaumont was able to observe the trapper's digestive processes; and the story of his experiments and observations, related in his book on the physiology of the digestion, is one of the most fascinating case histories in medicine. Beaumont fed him different types of food, to see how they were digested: beginning with

August 1 1825. At 12 o'clock I introduced through the perforation, into the stomach, the following articles of diet, suspended with a silk string, so as to pass in without pain: viz. a piece of high seasoned *á la mode beef*; a piece of *raw, salted fat pork*; a piece of *raw, salted, lean beef*; a piece of *boiled, salted beef*; a piece of *stale bread*; and a bunch of *raw, sliced cabbage*.

From time to time Beaumont withdrew the silk string, finding that the cabbage and the bread were digested first; then the pork and boiled beef. The *à la mode* beef was slower; and at lunchtime the raw beef, though slightly macerated on the surface, remained whole and entire. From numerous experiments of this nature Beaumont was able to show how the digestive processes worked: not through maceration, or putrefaction of foodstuff, but through the stomach dissolving them with the assistance of its acid supply.

The New Humoralism

The surprising revival of the period was humoralism – though it was not thought of as such, or spoken of by that name.

The most remarkable of the new humoralists, in that he accurately forecast by intuition what was to be confirmed by research a century later, was Théophile de Bordeu of Montpellier, a vitalist by inclination who worked, rather incongruously, in Paris at the court of Louis XV. De Bordeu suggested that certain organs of the body gave forth emanations, or secretions, which are absorbed in the bloodstream; and that health is dependent upon keeping the balance of these secretions – an idea that had come to him from observing the effects of castration.

This was speculative; but meanwhile in Padua – once so famous a breeding ground for famous anatomists, but by the eighteenth century sunk in obscurity – another researcher was putting forward the proposition which would eventually lead to the speculation being translated into physiological fact. Giovanni Morgagni had been appointed professor there in 1711; but it was not until after half a century of patient work that he published *De Sedibus et Causis Morborum*, five anatomical treatises in which he argued that diseases were entities related to specific bodily organs; that the symptoms reflected specific changes within these organs; and that if researchers spent less time worrying about abstractions like the archeus and got down to observing and analysing visible organic changes, they would be much more likely to find out the cause of diseases, and how to prevent or cure them.

It was not an entirely new idea – Erasistratus had held rather similar views;

Opposite: Il Ciarlatano by Pietro Longhi (1702–85)

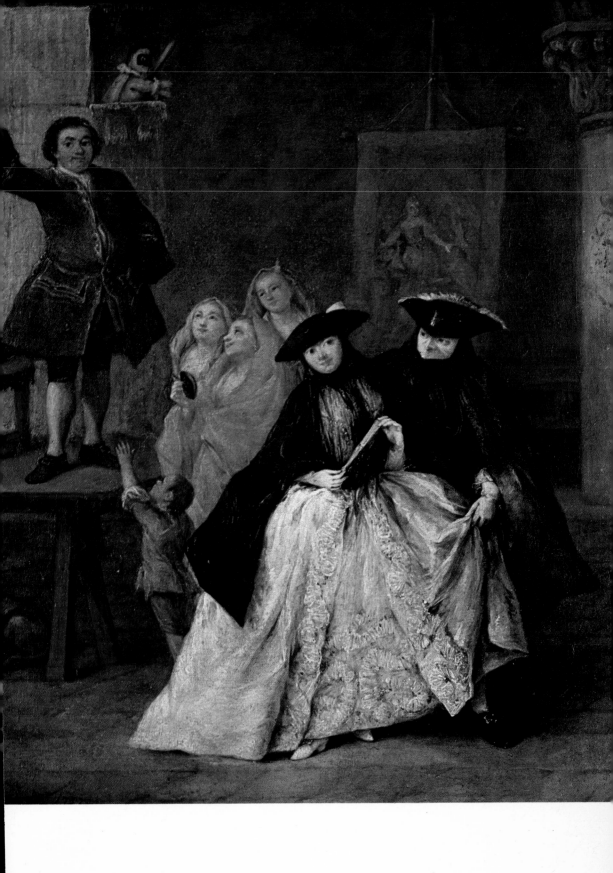

but it was new enough to make little immediate impact on the doctors of the time, involved as they were with their systems. Towards the end of the century, though, it attracted Xavier Bichat, and when he was appointed physician to the Hôtel Dieu in Paris in 1800, he set to work on it. Although a vitalist, his chief contribution to medicine came from his meticulous study of the organs of the body, and in particular their tissues. It was not, he came to the conclusion, the organs themselves, but their tissues which became diseased – sometimes even an individual tissue while the rest of the organ remained sound – like a plank of wood flawed by a knot. Bichat died young, but from his ideas, with the help of the microscope, it was a relatively easy step to the cellular pathology introduced by Theodor Schwann in the 1830s, later to be elaborated by Rudolf Virchow, and codified into the assertion 'there are no general diseases. From now on we shall recognise only diseases of organs and cells.'

This might have been taken as an indication that the humoral theory was finally superseded, and the basis of a new physiology laid. But Virchow himself was aware that there was more to it than that. 'Pathological anatomy and clinical work', he wrote,

although we fully recognise their justification and their independence, are the sources of new problems whose answers must be supplied by pathological physiology. Since these problems must for the most part be formulated by means of a laborious and comprehensive study of detailed phenomena in the sick, and upon the post-mortem table, we maintain that a precise and purposive development of anatomical and clinical experience is the most important requisite of the day. Through an empiricism of this sort there will gradually be brought into being a genuine theory of medicine.

So it turned out. While Virchow was working on his cellular pathology, his contemporary Claude Bernard was formulating a theory which was to give the old humoralism, and vitalism, a scientific basis.

Bernard made a great many contributions to physiology, and is generally regarded as the founder of experimental medicine – the study of artificially induced and controlled disease. The most important of them was his refinement of von Haller's theory about how the organs of the body work. The fundamental characteristic of living organisms, Bernard decided, is that they are able to maintain the constancy of their internal *milieu* – their internal environment. All the vital mechanisms, varied as they are, have only one object: that of preserving constant the conditions of life within the body. Man, for example, is constantly adapting himself internally to external changes; he may step out of cold air into a hot bath (or vice versa), yet his internal temperature will vary only marginally. It is this capacity of the body to maintain its equilibrium – later given the name 'homeostasis' by the Harvard physiologist Walter Cannon – which sets man free to achieve his full development; in ordinary circumstances, he does not often have to worry about making adjustments to deal with the perpetual changes in his external environment, except to put on a coat when he goes out. But when his homeostat breaks down, he falls ill; he has to begin to think about his physical functioning, and find out how to set it to right, again.

Bernard's thesis suggested that many of the ideas of the systematists, and even the old humoral theory, had not been simply wild and ill-considered guesses (as by this time they were considered); they could be seen as intuitive gropings towards an essential truth. In particular, Bernard revealed the essential correctness of the idea that there was a link between the body fluids and psychological characteristics or manifestations. As his biographers, J. and E. Olmstead noted, when Bernard gave a lecture at the Sorbonne on the physiology of the heart, he refused to take up the strictly mechanistic attitude of the heart as a pump: instead

he undertook to justify the association of the word 'heart' in literature and common speech with the emotions. He pointed out that although the characteristic movement of the heart is the earliest as well as the latest manifestation of life, and is independent of nervous stimulus, nevertheless the nervous system exercises a negative control over its beating . . . A strong nerve stimulus, such as may be provoked by terror or deep emotion, will stop the heart long enough to prevent the arrival of blood in the brain, and the result will be fainting. A milder stimulus will stop the heart more briefly, imperceptibly except to the physiologist, but the function will be resumed with an increase of tempo, fluttering, or palpitation, which will send more blood to the brain, and result in a blush.

Bernard went on to relate his own physical disorders to emotional disturbances – blaming his digestive troubles on his country's disgraceful defeat in the war of 1870; and he included man's emotional characteristics as well as his constitution and physical condition in his concept of the 'terrain' in which diseases germinate. To Bernard, ill-health was ordinarily an indication that the body's homeostatic mechanism had broken down, and that therefore it was failing to deal expeditiously, as it normally would, with disease agents. The logical extension of this theory was that in cases of ill-health the search should be directed to finding out not merely which disease agent was responsible, but why the homeostat was not performing its task of resisting it – a diagnosis which could have important consequences for treatment: in his own case, for example, the homeostat had been disrupted because of shame and anger over France's humiliation – not because of something toxic he had eaten. But while Bernard was perfecting his thesis of the importance of the terrain, his friend and colleague Louis Pasteur was busy examining the habits of microbial agents of disease; and in the excitement caused by his discoveries, the significance of Bernard's hypothesis was missed.

The other re-establisher of the humoral theory was Bernard's eccentric contemporary, Charles Brown-Séquard, born in Mauritius and a restless pursuer of scientific truth in America, France, Britain and Switzerland, never able to stay in one place for long. He might have done more effective research if he had been less frenetic – but on the other hand he might not have dared to attempt what he did.

Bernard had described the *milieu interieur*, regulated by its homeostatic mechanism; Brown-Séquard found out how the homeostat worked, through the secretions of the ductless glands. In the 1880s he injected himself with fluid from the testes of guinea pigs, and then in due course presented himself to the Société de Biologie to show how the treatment had taken twenty years off his age. It is impossible to tell whether this feat was accomplished by the injections or by auto-suggestion; and although Serge Voronoff, using testicular transplants from monkeys, and Eugen Steinach, employing surgical operations for rejuvenation purposes, were both to claim highly successful results, the idea has since fallen out of favour. Brown-Séquard's reputation is not unchallenged; but he is conceded to have earned the title of founder of endocrinology. He understood the intricacies of the nervous system, Harley Williams claimed:

as few men of his time did; he divined that among those delicate fibres, those cells and ganglions of the brain and spinal cord, there played the eternal rivers of the circulating blood which brought chemicals to stimulate or to soothe the sensitive nerves. He discovered, or confirmed, a secret which many before him had guessed; namely, that we move our limbs, live our emotions, and think our

131

thoughts through a complex but very beautiful mechanism that lies between nerve tendrils so fine as to be invisible, and fluid secretions that are powerful yet beyond the reach of chemistry.

But the work of Brown-Séquard, and of Bernard, was not at the time fully appreciated; and they were to be overshadowed by Pasteur.

10

MODERN TIMES

The Doctor and the Quack

NOBODY has yet been able to account satisfactorily for the astonishing revolution that took place in medicine in the middle of the nineteenth century, and is generally linked with Pasteur. Most of the changes that were to take place had been forecast or foreshadowed by earlier theorists; but it needed someone, or something, to bring them to fruition. Presumably the industrial revolution and the spread of democratic institutions helped to provide the required economic, social and political environment; whatever the reason, most branches of medicine shared in the advance. Each branch of medicine, though, made its advances separately; and before going on to examine them, it is as well to take a look at how the medical profession settled down into its present form. For centuries, the physicians had done their best to obtain a guild status; they had managed to lay down standards and draw up regulations, but had lacked consistent success in imposing them. In the nineteenth century they were at last to be given the powers they needed to enforce their decisions, and to learn how to use them.

The story of the development of a professional ethic ought to be inspiring; but its most obvious characteristics were envy, malice and uncharitableness – and it was not only heretical individuals who suffered. From medieval times, the different clinical groupings and factions had fought each other with remarkable consistent ferocity and malice.

The war between the physicians – who thought of themselves as the only true doctors – and the surgeons had been particularly venomous. Their rivalry was already established by the thirteenth century, when Henry de Mondeville described how a physician behaved when he found that he had a surgical case on his hands. Surgeons (he would tell the patient) were either ignorant, or, if they knew anything, they had learned it from physicians; they were also clumsy and avaricious. The patients, hearing this, would probably beg the physician to perform the operation himself. But if he still demanded to go to a surgeon, the physician would take good care to recommend one he knew to be incompetent. As for the surgeon – de Mondeville went on – he could be just as crafty, assuring the patient that physicians might be great talkers but when it came down to actual remedies, all they could prescribe was useless purgatives.

The division between physicians and surgeons was, in theory at least, reasonably well-defined by what treatment they gave: the physician using his drugs; the surgeon his knife. More galling to the physician, therefore, was the existence of men styling themselves physicians, but without the university qualifications which had come to be considered as indispensable by those physicians who possessed them. These interlopers were of two main types: clerics, who sometimes used Christian methods of healing, but might practise other forms of medicine, and apothecaries, who occupied a position midway between the chemist and the general practitioner of today.

The physicians were most successful in establishing their monopoly in Britain, where Thomas Linacre, court physician to King Henry VIII, persuaded him to grant a licence for a self-perpetuating professional body – the prototype of many: the College of Physicians of London. His biographer, John Freind, later described how Linacre:

saw in how low a condition the practice of physic then was, that it was mostly engrossed by illiterate monks and empirics, who in an infamous manner imposed on the public – the Bishop of London or the Dean of St Paul's having the power of approving or admitting the practitioners in London, and the rest of the bishops in their several dioceses. And he found there was no way left of redressing his grievance, but by giving encouragement to men of reputation and learning, and placing this power of licensing in more proper hands. Upon these motives he projected the foundation of our College; and using his interest at court, particularly with that great patriot and munificent promoter of all learning, Cardinal Wolsey, he procured letters patent from the king which were confirmed by parliament to establish a corporate society of physicians in this city, by virtue of which authority the college, as a corporation now enjoys the sole privilege of admitting all persons whatsoever to the practice of physic, as well as that of supervising all prescriptions.

The aims were worthy; but as soon as they had established their quasi-monopoly, the physicians began to consolidate it by using their powers against all potential rivals; clerics, surgeons, apothecaries and chemists who dared to treat patients. The Guild of Physicians – for this was in effect what Linacre had contrived to found – immediately instituted restrictive practices, limiting the number of doctors and so enabling them to charge inflated fees. They were able to do this on what sounded the plausible excuse that only Oxford or Cambridge graduates could be recognised as having the required qualifications. But their attempts to suppress rivals were unsuccessful; largely because in the sixteenth century the surgeons, though still not highly regarded, began to enjoy a greater measure of respect, because that gunpowder had so stimulated the demand for their services.

As we have seen, though, no sooner had the surgeons managed to free themselves from control by the physicians than they began to discriminate against their own rivals. The surgeons proper, contemptuous of the mere barbers who practised surgery as an adjunct of their trade, sought powers to prevent them doing so. Like the physicians, the surgeons could put forward what appeared to be sound arguments for giving them the powers they asked for. Only thus, they claimed, could the public be protected from untrained and fraudulent practitioners. Disconcertingly often, though, the ranks of the untrained threw up a Paré, far more skilful than his more highly qualified colleagues. Paré himself broke through the prejudice; others were crushed by it. A century later the Franciscan Frère Jacques perfected the technique of removing gallstones, and successfully demonstrated it before the medical faculty in Paris. They could have forgiven failure, but that he should have performed it better than they could was too much: Frère Jacques was hounded out, and after his death, it was asserted, even his name was erased from tombstone and records, to prevent respect being paid to his memory.

In much the same way, physicians found themselves constantly at war with the apothecaries. Apothecaries had originally been chemists: they owed their elevation in certain countries chiefly to the reluctance of the physician, once he had qualified, to waste his time on general practice. For the needy, to call in a physician was an expensive business – particularly as he usually prescribed expensive drugs. The local apothecary, though, was often prepared to make visits; and he made up his own prescriptions, which was cheaper.

The chief complaint about apothecaries was that they cheated the patient by prescribing bogus drugs: as they made their prescriptions up themselves the temptation must often have been too much for them. On the Continent, following the Hohenstaufen principle, the distinction between chemist and doctor was generally upheld – even though it could not always be enforced. But in Britain the apothecaries managed to entrench themselves as general practitioners, in spite of the powerful attacks mounted on them. At the beginning of the eighteenth century a court case established their right to treat as well as dispense; and by the beginning of the nineteenth they had formed their own association, for which they obtained state recognition, rights, privileges and disciplinary powers.

Characteristically, as soon as they had secured their nest the apothecaries set about feathering it. Anguished cries went up from doctors trained in Edinburgh and Dublin (many of them much better trained, at that time, than the English product) arriving in England: the upstart apothecaries' association was refusing to allow them to practise unless they qualified for an English licence, which could be troublesome and expensive. Inevitably, too, the apothecaries, having successfully made the transition from chemists to doctors, determined to prevent the chemists from following their example. They tried to secure disciplinary control over the chemists, as well as over their own members; but the attempt was a failure.

The apothecaries, however, were lucky in that they acquired status just in time to be recognised as doctors, when the various and previously disunited elements of the medical profession began to coagulate into a profession. How uncertain their status had been can be gauged from Thackeray's *Pendennis*:

There were those alive who remembered having seen his name painted on a board, which was surmounted by a gilt pestle and mortar over the door of a very humble little shop in the city of Bath, where Mr Pendennis exercised the profession of apothecary and surgeon; and where he not only attended gentlemen in their sickrooms, and ladies at the most interesting periods in their lives, but would condescend to sell a brown paper plaster to a farmer's wife across the counter – or to vend toothbrushes, hair powder and London perfumery.

Pendennis, though, was an exception: 'that little apothecary who sold a stray customer a pennyworth of salts, or a more fragrant cake of Windsor soap, was a gentleman of good education, and of as old a family as any in the whole country of Somerset.' He had become an apothecary because his father had died insolvent; and as soon as opportunity offered he quit his

Surgery and Hospitals

Primitive ambulance used in Portugal in the nineteenth century to transport the sick to hospital

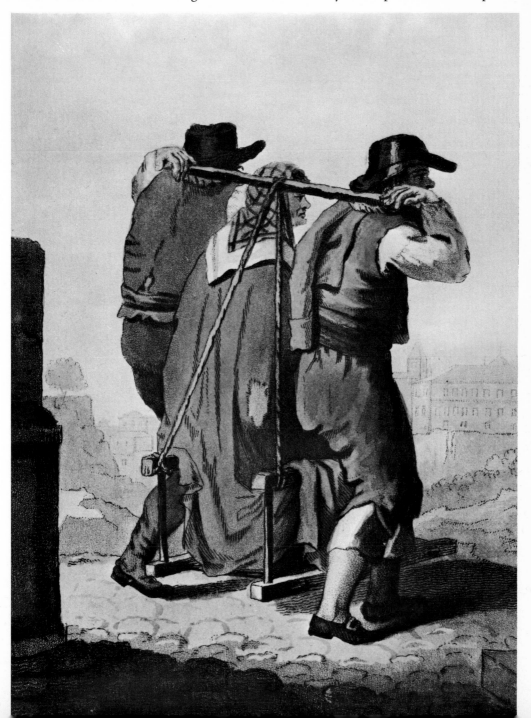

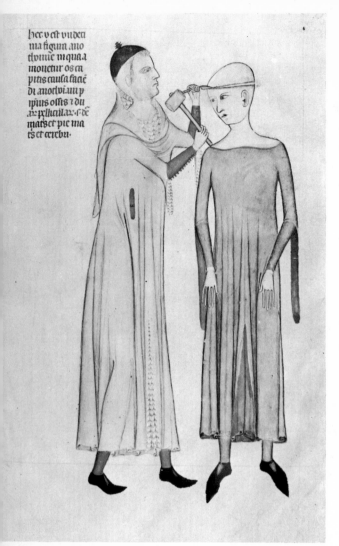

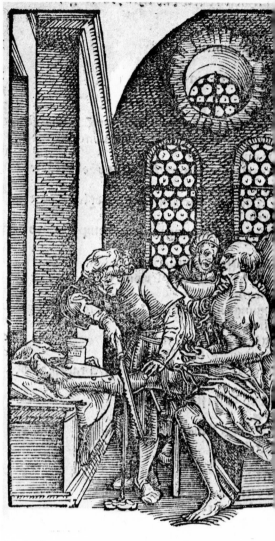

Left: Medieval surgeon performing an operation on the skull. From a manuscript on Galenic anatomy

Right: Amputation, from Paracelsus' *Surgery* (1549). Paracelsus recommended the use of anaesthetics for operations of this kind

Opposite page. Above: Two illustrations from a seventeenth-century work showing the first intravenous injection, used for anaesthetic purposes; and blood transfusions from dog to man and from man to man

Below: Illustration from Beaumont's *Experiments and Observations* (1838) showing the digestive system visible through a hole in the stomach of a trapper, who had been accidentally shot

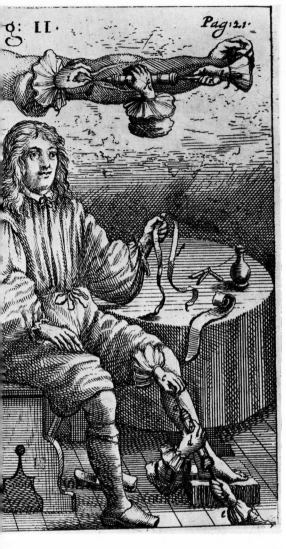

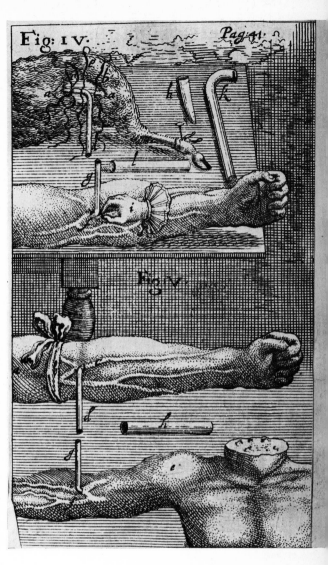

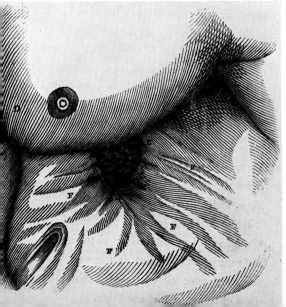

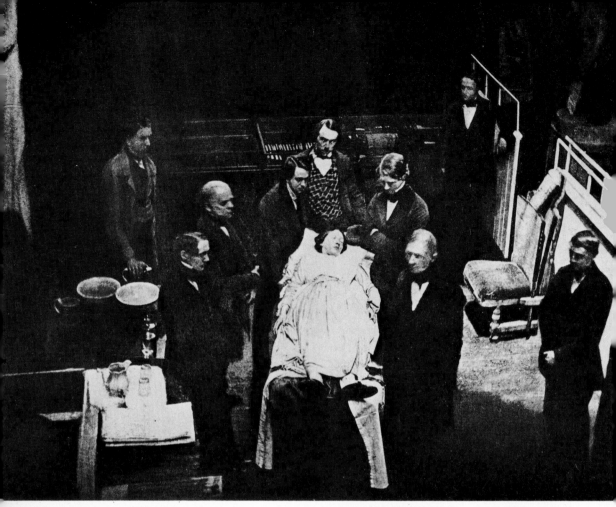

Operation in Massachusetts
General Hospital in the winter of
1847, using ether as the anaesthetic,
as introduced by William Morton
the previous year; showing Dr
Warren and his colleagues

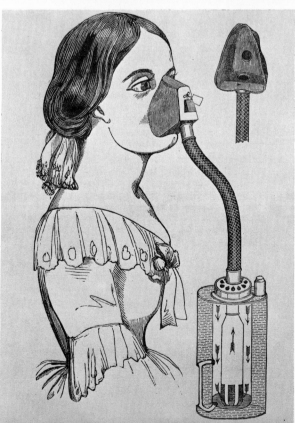

Administration of chloroform in
the 1850s—a more effective, though
less safe anaesthetic than ether

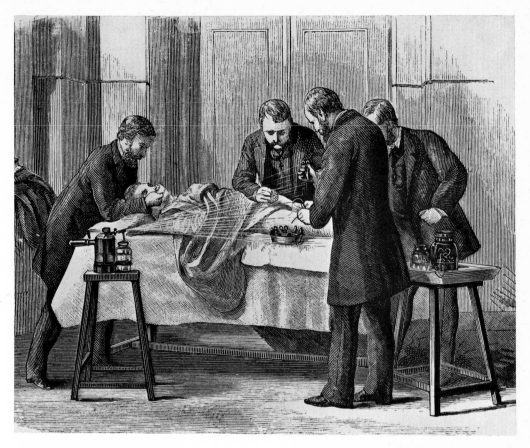

Use of Joseph Lister's carbolic spray, the first effective step in antiseptic surgery, in an operation about 1880

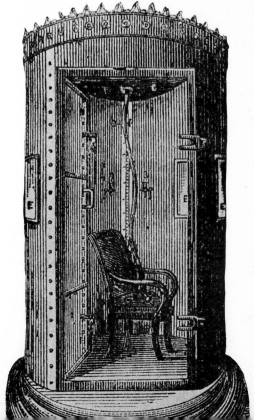

Compressed air *cloche* for dental operations (*c.* 1880), one of the earliest applications of anaesthesia to dentistry

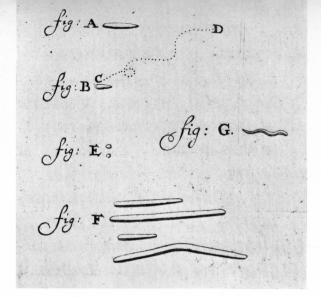

First pictures of bacteria, seen under
the microscope and described by
the Dutch scientist Leeuwenhoek
in the seventeenth century

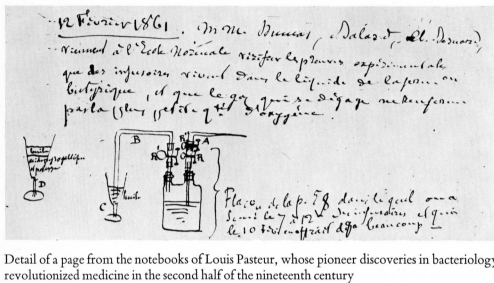

Detail of a page from the notebooks of Louis Pasteur, whose pioneer discoveries in bacteriology
revolutionized medicine in the second half of the nineteenth century

Florence Nightingale in the hospital at Scutari. Miss Nightingale not only reformed the nursing
profession, but also transformed standards of hygiene and cleanliness in hospitals

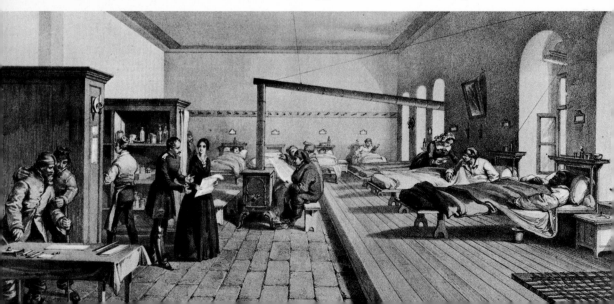

Photograph taken in 1862 showing
early medical use of electricity by
Duchenne de Boulogne. Such
experiments were particularly
valuable for the development of
nerve-surgery

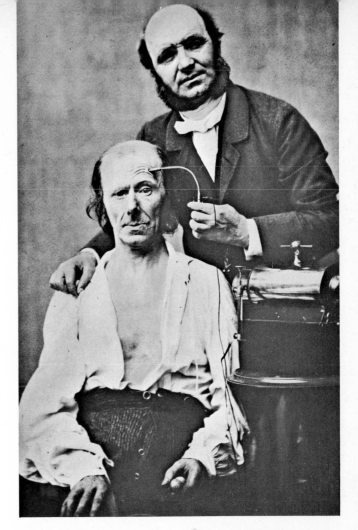

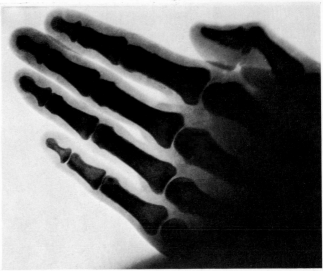

X-ray photograph of a hand made
in 1896, one of the earliest X-rays
to be made in Great Britain

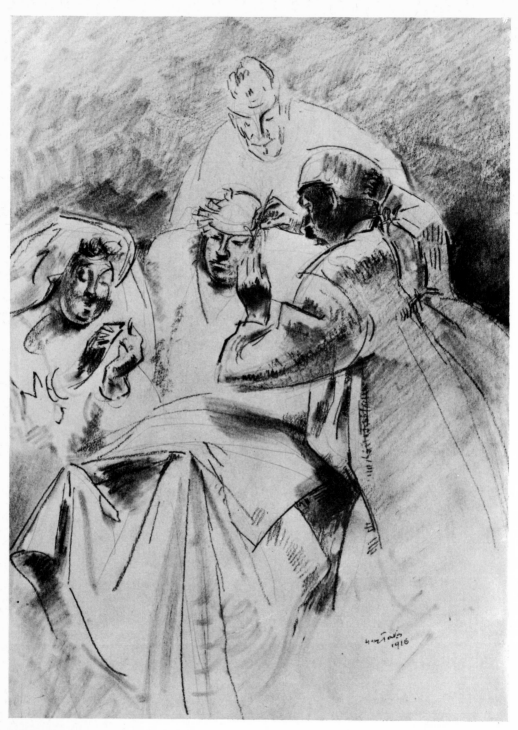

The Birth of Plastic Surgery (1916) by Henry Tonks. The artist was trained as a surgeon and returned to practice during the 1914–18 war. The figure on the patient's left is a self-portrait

shop to become a family doctor. To the physicians, the idea of a doctor qualifying through peddling pills was disgraceful; and they did their best to secure the exclusion of the apothecaries from professional status by objecting that they had no academic qualifications. But although by this time the medical schools could claim to have improved their teaching, in view of what was taught at them the apothecary's chief asset was that he had *not* attended them.

This was particularly true of medicine in the US in the eighteenth and early nineteenth century. Low though standards were, they were probably higher than in Europe; at least doctors there learned by experience – an admirable teacher, if they had any powers of observation; whereas medical students in Europe learned largely by rote, and what they were taught was largely incorrect. Osler believed the average American doctor in Colonial times was less cruel and probably much more effective than his European counterpart; and Sigerist, agreeing, pointed out that the practical training had a further advantage: no hard and fast distinction was possible between medicine, surgery and other specialities. The American country doctor, rough and ready though his methods were, may often have deserved the halo that tradition and Westerns have given him.

But in the United States, as in every country, established doctors were obsessed by the nagging fear of outsiders; of quacks. Why – the qualified doctor understandably asked himself – should his training count for nothing, as it might when any charlatan could put up his plate, and even advertise for patients? The same arguments that Linacre had used to secure a charter for qualified physicians came into use again in favour of the setting up of an enclosed medical profession, embracing only those who had qualifications, and having powers not only to exclude the unqualified, but also to prevent them from practising.

The campaign to create a single, unified profession had varying degrees of success in different countries. In France, orthodoxy persuaded the State to enact and enforce a code designed to prevent unqualified practitioners from treating patients; and some states of the US adopted similar rules. In Britain, however, there was more tenderness for the liberty of the subject. Nobody, it was argued, should be prevented from treating patients, so long as he did not do so under false pretences, pretending he was qualified. Doctors alone should be allowed to prescribe certain drugs, and to treat patients in hospitals; but no man should be penalised for treating patients simply because he was not a member of the profession, unless he pretended to be.

Whether or not there was active persecution of unqualified practitioners, the dividing line between members of the profession and 'quacks' quickly hardened; and not to the advantage of the public. It became difficult for the profession, once established, to absorb newcomers, as it had in the past – first surgeons, then apothecaries. And some of the groups left outside were a loss to the profession: notably the manipulators.

Bonesetting had long been a craft practised chiefly by men who happened to have the gift, or who had learned the craft through apprenticeship to someone who had it. Although a few bonesetters had become nationally famous (or notorious), as a group they had not aspired to professional dignity. But now, they were actually excluded: doctors who sent their patients to a bonesetter, however skilful they might know him to be, risked disciplinary action for entrusting them to a quack. In the 1860s, shortly after the Act had been passed conferring monopolistic status on the medical profession in Britain, Sir James Paget warned his colleagues that it was no use condemning bonesetters, or the people who went to them, if doctors could not do the required manipulation themselves. But as manipulation was not included in the curriculum, the field was left clear, as Paget feared, for the unqualified.

At first, doctors were inclined to dismiss such warnings. Bonesetting, after all, was not so extensive to constitute a serious threat to their professional monopoly. But at this point – in much the same way as the apothecaries had filled the vacuum left by the physicians when they had acquired their monopoly – the practitioners of a new therapeutic system, based on bonesetting, began to evolve.

A Virginian, Andrew Taylor Still, found that his technique of spinal manipulation appeared to cure patients of all manner of disorders, from gallstones to worms; he evolved the theory that spinal lesions, small deviations from the normal articulation, were the cause of disease, and that manipulation, to put them back into place, was consequently the cure. A few years later, in a different part of the US, Daniel Palmer came to a similar conclusion. Both collected disciples around them: Still's called themselves osteopaths; Palmer's, chiropractors. The results might have been due largely to suggestion, but that they were often beneficial was indisputable; and both systems began to attract patients, first in the US and later in European countries. Osteopathic and chiropractic training colleges were opened, with curricula of their own; and in spite of some savage persecution by orthodoxy, both survived and flourished, taking over many of the functions of the old family doctor.

It was no coincidence that Christian healing also began a revival in the second half of the nineteenth century. The new professional orthodoxy was basically materialist: and this left many patients, and not only Christians, with a sense of deprivation. But the Churches, Catholic or Protestant, were not the beneficiaries. The reason, Guirdham suggested in his *The Nature of Healing*, is that 'distrust of mysticism seems to be at its worst in Christianity'. As soon as the Catholic Church developed an administrative superstructure, it began to regard mystical or supernatural experience as something dangerous, partly because it was outside administrative control, partly because it suggested ordinary men and women might have a short cut to God that was denied to priests and even to Popes. Where healing could not be suppressed it was regulated, as at Lourdes; but on the whole the Church's attitude was mistrustful. The Anglicans became even more hostile, leaning towards rationalism; and although Wesley came near to regarding his work as a healing mission, as Jesus's had been, his followers also drifted away from the idea.

In the nineteenth century several new cults arose to remedy this spiritual deficiency, the most successful being Christian Science. Its origins were curious. The United States had had its share of magnetisers, the most celebrated of them being Elisha Perkins, a contemporary of Mesmer's. Perkins had been a country doctor, and in his rounds had noticed the muscular contractions experienced by some patients when touched with a metal rod. This, apparently, gave him the idea for his 'metallic tractors', which he brought out just before the end of the century; small metal nails or skewers with which he stroked the patient's body much as Greatrax had done – always from the centre outwards, as if to stroke away the pain. The fact that he put the tractors on sale, however, got him into trouble with the Connecticut Medical Society, which expelled him; and after a few years the craze for the tractors – they had enjoyed a substantial sale at about £10 the pair – began to fall off. Perkins thereupon tried to restore his fortunes with the help of a yellow fever cure; but he died of the disease before the cure had time to catch on – a fate that naturally did not restore confidence in his tractors, though his son had with their assistance enjoyed a lucrative visit to England.

Magnetiser-mesmerists, however, continued to go the rounds in the United States; one of them aroused the interest of a Maine watchmaker, Phineas Quimby; Quimby became a mesmerist himself; and it was a patient of his in the 1860s who later, as Mary Baker Eddy, became the founder of Christian Science. Mrs Eddy was later to repudiate Quimby; but she had already adopted those of his ideas which accorded with her own in her *Science and Health*. Her theory was vitalist: that healing is a spiritual process, operating through the divine mind, from which the human mind can draw inspiration and thereupon health, with truth and love as the therapeutic agents. The method was an interesting development from Mesmer's, designed to liberate the imagination, to enable it to play on health, and in spite of the quirks of its founder, Christian Science quickly established itself.

Other forms of healing caught on towards the end of the nineteenth century, including spiritualism; which, when it shed its preoccupation with the souls of the dead in the next world, and began to concentrate on the health of its members in this one, began to attract a wider following. Individual Christian healers, working as Jesus had done, also made reputations for themselves in many parts of the world; so that in the twentieth century, healing began to enjoy an unexpected revival.

The only unorthodox system of medicine, in fact, to suffer defeat in its contest with orthodoxy was homeopathy. Partly this was due to its failure to provide convincing proof that the microdose worked; but a more telling reason was the reluctance of its practitioners to resist orthodoxy's encroachments. In order to maintain their status as doctors, they allowed members of the profession in the US and Britain to infiltrate, and eventually to take over, the homeopathic hospitals. Only in France, where they were less accommodating (the running battle with orthodoxy appeared to act as a stimulus) did they continue to flourish.

The unification of the qualified practitioners of medicine into a single profession, then, did not have the desired result of promoting orthodoxy; it simply meant that rival practices grew up and flourished alongside. It did not even have the effect of imposing orthodoxy within the profession. The aim had never been to compel all doctors to conform to a single pattern of treatment – it was always realised that an individual practitioner would have, and should be encouraged to have, his own views on how to handle specific disorders or specific patients; but it was hoped that a damper would be put on the kind of clinical fads and fashions which had been initiated or exploited by unscrupulous practitioners, because the profession was unable to discipline them. As things turned out, it still couldn't. Once a man (or a woman – women soon fought their way into the profession; the work of Florence Nightingale, though she was not a doctor, made it difficult to continue arguing that they were unfitted for such work) had qualified, he could employ eccentric and sometimes bogus treatments, if they happened to be profitable, with relative impunity. And fashions in treatment, and even in disease, continued to attract the profession when it was established.

The last of the old-styled systematists had been the Breton, François Broussais, who in Napoleonic times advanced a variation of the 'tonus' theory. There were no specific diseases, he insisted; the difference between symptoms merely reflected the degree of excessive (or inadequate) excitation. But he went further: the first symptom of disease, he believed, was inflammation – the body's reaction to irritation; and the cause of the disturbance was usually to be found in the digestive system: gastro-enteritis. All treatment, therefore, should be directed at the stomach, regardless of where the symptoms manifested themselves. Although Broussais ended up as Professor of Pathology at the Paris Academy of Medicine, his doctrines were already being eroded in his lifetime, and were demolished by the work of Bernard and Pasteur; yet their simplicity continued to attract doctors. The vogue for 'Colitis', so vividly described by Axel Munthe in *The Story of San Michele* ('a new disease was dumped on the market, a new word was coined, a gold coin indeed, Colitis! It was a neat complaint safe from the surgeon's knife, always at hand when wanted, suitable to everybody's taste') was a tribute to the staying-power of Broussais' idea; so was Metchnikoff's thesis that health and longevity could be secured by introducing a kind of bacteriological police force into the digestive tract. There have been several variants recently, some popular with surgeons: Bernard Shaw's satirical study of the surgeon Cutler Walpole, with his habit of treating all patients for blood poisoning by cutting out the 'nuciform sac', had a grotesque echo a few years later when the idea of disease being caused by 'focal sepsis' led to numbers of patients suffering from undiagnosed disorders having all their teeth pulled out. If an unqualified practitioner had adumbrated the theory it would have been dismissed with ridicule; yet because it spread within the profession, it was tolerated, and thousands of patients became its victims.

Even more disturbing, though, than the continuance of old deplorable clinical failings was the growth of arbitrary divisions within the medical profession. For the convenience of educators and administrators, the trend set in towards specialisation. Lecturers at medical schools might refer to the need to keep the 'whole man' in mind, but anatomy, biology, psychiatry, botany and the rest were usually taught as if they were independent unrelated subjects. After graduation, too, specialisation became dominant, with students who had impressed examiners dividing up not merely into physicians and surgeons, but into even narrower and more self-contained groups concentrating on a particular type of disease, or a particular organ of the body.

But this trend was utterly out of key with the needs of patients. The discoveries of the endocrinologists had suggested that the future of medicine lay in discovering more about why the body's homeostatic system went out of order, and how to prevent it from doing so, rather than worrying overmuch about the end product – the symptoms. But once specialisation in individual sets of symptoms (or individual organs) had begun it proved impossible to reverse. By the 1960s this was beginning to cause concern. As the Oxford botanist Professor C. D. Darlington pointed out, if the evolutionary theory is accepted, then, as Darwin had shown, 'cats eating mice, mice eating bees, and bees pollinating clover act as a single chain of vital and varying reactions . . . similarly we know that when an animal eats a plant the process concerns botany as much as zoology, medicine as much as agriculture, ecology as much as physiology. We now see that all are connected.' But in medical research, Darlington complained, they have become disconnected, fragmented:

Outside the universities this process leads to specialised establishments for research where all inquiry is supposedly directed to a particular branch of agriculture or medicine; where a man may be committed to devote all his life to study the effects on the body of one kind of disease or one kind of radiation. Inside the universities this process leads to a break up of education. The university is being brought down to the level of the polytechnic. And our culture has already been shattered, not into two fragments, but into twenty or more.

One of the fundamental weaknesses of the specialist approach was described by Professor Albert Szent-Gyorgi:

More than twenty years ago I felt I had enough experience to be able to tackle a complex biological problem. I chose motion, that is, the function of muscle. My laboratory was soon able to isolate from muscle two sorts of molecules, which could be described in the language of classical chemistry, and which, if put together in the right order, formed something like an artificial muscle, which could move outside the body and could thus be analysed with the current methods. I was convinced that within a matter of weeks we would completely understand how muscle generates motion. Then I worked for twenty years without making progress. One important point I overlooked was 'organisation'.

'Organisation' means that if nature puts two things together in a meaningful way, something new is generated which cannot be described, any more, in terms of the qualities of its constituents. This is true through the whole gamut of complexity, from atomic nuclei and electrons up to macromolecules or a complex individual. Nature is not additive. If this is true, then the opposite is also true, and when I take two things apart I have thrown away something, something which has been the very essence of that system, of that level of organisation.

– but if nature was not additive, then most of the specialist research in progress was futile: it might lead to refinements of what was already known, but it could not throw light on the unknown.

Specialism was also damaging to the doctors themselves. The old-style general physician or surgeon ceased to exist. William Osler, who died in 1919, was perhaps the last of them; a man in the Sydenham/Boerhaave tradition, with catholic interests and a way of inspiring his students. Like Boerhaave, Osler had originally intended to follow his Canadian father into the ministry; but changed his mind, became a medical student and, after doing a kind of medical Grand Tour of Europe came back to America to become, in a remarkably short space of time, the best known member of his profession. He wrote what was to become the most widely read of all textbooks, and one of the most engaging of all histories of medicine; he was acknowledged to be a brilliant clinician; and he did some important scientific research. But as Sigerist emphasised, his achievements do not account for his renown, which 'depends upon his personality as physician, as teacher, as man'.

Osler himself realised that he could not have become what he was if he had simply been a physician. Again and again in his lectures he returned to the theme of the need for the doctor to treat himself (as well as his patients) as a whole man: 'while medicine is to be your vocation,' he told students, 'or calling, see to it that you also have an avocation – some intellectual pastime

143

which may serve to keep you in touch with the world of art, of science or of letters.' Yet even as he was lecturing, medicine was congealing into those watertight compartments which too often cut off the specialist, not merely from other branches of medicine, but from wider interests.

The extinction of the Osler-style doctor was illustrated in the *Times* in the summer of 1964. The headline described the deceased as 'a distinguished surgeon', who had had the unusual honour of having been President of both the Royal College of Surgeons and the British Medical Association. But, the obituarist went on, 'he was in some ways typical of many surgeons of his generation [he had been a medical student at the turn of the century, when Osler's influence was at its peak] in that he avoided taking the final steps to limit his field of surgical activity. He remained a general surgeon, and he was therefore perhaps less well known internationally in the branch of surgery in which he was especially interested than some of his contemporaries in the same field who had made the decision to be complete specialists.' 'Perhaps less well known' was putting it charitably; a general surgeon could no longer hope to count for much in a faculty dominated by specialists; the chance of another Osler emerging had become slender.

Anaesthetics and Asepsis

Within the profession, though, in the latter part of the nineteenth century, the most spectacular advance was made by surgeons. By mid-century they had managed to establish themselves alongside, though still a little below, the physicians; but there was no prospect of surgery improving its status further unless it could exorcise two ever-present spectres: the pain felt by patients while the operation was in progress and often after it; and the risk of death from infection.

Civilised man's prolonged failure to find ways to remove or reduce pain presents what is surely the most baffling problem in medical history. That certain plants could be prescribed as pain-killers was known to primitive tribes. Opium was in use as early as the third millennium BC. The narcotic effects of Indian hemp were known in ancient times in the East; and surgeons were using it in China before operations in the second century AD. Alcohol also came to be used for this purpose: a Persian writer in the tenth century AD

Opposite: Two French cartoons, *c.* 1800, attacking the new fashion for vaccination

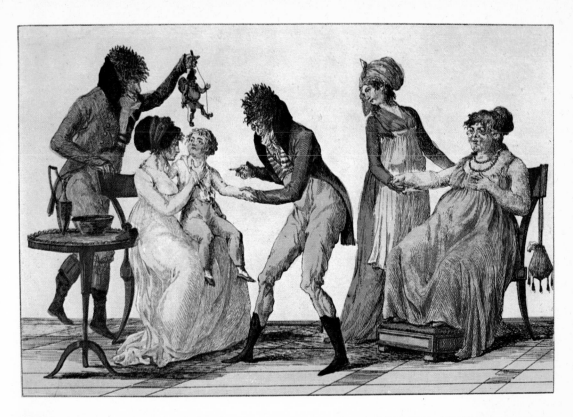

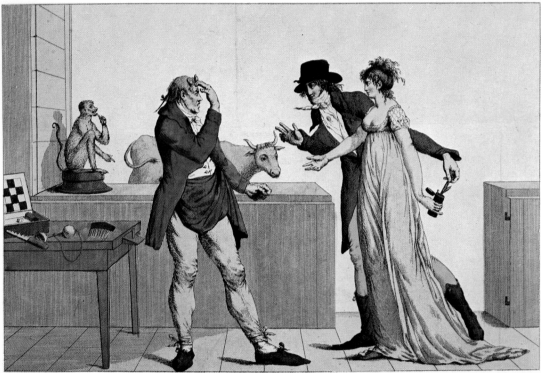

described how women about to undergo caesarians were 'bemused' with wine.

Stories of the use of drugs to put people to sleep from a variety of motives abound in medieval times. Michael Scot left a prescription for surgeons:

Take of opium, mandragora and henbane equal parts, pound and mix them with water. When you want to saw or cut a man, dip a rag in this and put it to his nostrils. He will soon sleep so deep that you may do what you wish.

It is true that, as one researcher caustically put it, many of the sleep-inducers prescribed in the Middle Ages, 'do not make even a guinea pig nod'. But the point was that they made human beings nod – whether through suggestion, or by some now forgotten means, is not known. They were still in use – or at least vividly remembered – during the Renaissance: Shakespeare made several references to the use of sleep-inducing drugs ('not poppy, not mandragora, not all the drowsy spirits of the world, shall ever medicine thee to that sweet sleep'), and Paracelsus popularised laudanum, a tincture of opium. Yet by the eighteenth century a patient about to be operated on was lucky if he received anything to kill the pain. He might deliberately make himself drunk, but this did not always work satisfactorily – and was not liked by some surgeons.

What makes the story still more puzzling is that highly intelligent men continued to 'discover' anaesthesia, and realise its potential value in medicine without making any real effort to publicise or exploit it. Shortly before the end of the eighteenth century Humphry Davy, examining the effect of nitrous oxide on animals, was so struck by it that he plucked up the courage to try the gas on himself – and later on his friends, the poets Coleridge and Wordsworth. They were much impressed by the ability of the gas to remove pain; and Davy actually suggested that it could 'probably be used to advantage in surgical operations'. The proposal was ignored; and Davy reverted to his chemistry. A few years later his assistant, Faraday, again demonstrated the pain-killing effects of nitrous oxide; still to no purpose.

Also in the early part of the nineteenth century, it was discovered that mesmerism could be used to remove the pain of operations; but unluckily, not until after it had appeared to be thoroughly discredited. Part of the reason for this was that Mesmer himself had not succeeded in differentiating between the varieties of trance state; and some of his followers were led into confusion as a consequence. The unluckiest was John Elliotson, the doctor who had been responsible for introducing the stethoscope into Britain, and the first holder of a medical professorship at London University. Becoming convinced of the therapeutic potential of mesmerism, Elliotson began to demonstrate it before London audiences – the public being allowed in: Dickens and Tom Moore attended – and Thackeray, who was to dedicate *Esmond* to him. But like Mesmer, Elliotson was thinking in terms of magnetism, which was to involve him in easily disproven assertions about the power of objects into which he had induced – as he thought – animal magnetism. In any case, as some of his subjects happened to be hysterics, the trances which they went into and their behaviour in them had more affinity to spiritualism than to what was later to be practised as hypnosis. As a result his enemies – already convinced that he was a dangerous radical by the fact that he wore trousers and sidewhiskers instead of the conventional garb of the physician of the period – joined forces against him. In 1838 he was told to stop his exhibitions; and he resigned his Chair.

A few years later, when tempers had died down, Elliotson was asked to give the Harveian Oration in connection with the bicentenary of Harvey's death. He took the opportunity to break with tradition once again by giving it in English, rather than in Latin; and he devoted a part of it to recalling the ridicule with which Harvey's colleagues had greeted the theory of the circulation of the blood. But this was small consolation for his failure to persuade the profession that mesmerism was worth investigating; particularly as that failure had only confirmed them in their assumption that it was spurious. Elliotson's tragedy, as Harley Williams commented in a sympathetic appraisal, 'was that he recognised the psychological wireless but was always searching for the wires', and as his search happened to be fruitless, he brought only discredit to the broadcasting system. Consequently even when hypnotism was laboriously disentangled from mesmerism, it was also suspect – and to some extent has remained so until the present day.

There was some justification for the scepticism of Elliotson's colleagues; but there was none for their refusal to take seriously the work of James Esdaile, the first man to exploit mesmerism specifically for the purpose of putting patients to sleep so that he could operate on them painlessly. Esdaile happened to be unusually well placed to experiment with it, as he was employed by the East India Company, who were not inclined to worry greatly about how he treated their coolies so long as he cured them and got them back to work. As for the patients, astonished to find that he was able to operate on them painlessly, they were not likely to object; and although there were attacks on Esdaile in the Indian medical journals, there was no resident medical Establishment at hand powerful enough to intervene.

It is difficult to exaggerate the potential importance of Esdaile's work. He performed hundreds of serious operations under mesmeric trance, including amputations, and thousands of minor ones, painlessly and with a negligible fatality rate; and he did enough work with hypnosis on mental and nervous disorders to realise that the prospects were encouraging for them, too. But while he was in mid-career, chloroform appeared as a counter-attraction; and although he was able to show that his method of inducing anaesthesia was decidedly safer, the prejudice against it was strong enough to lead to its re-placement by inhalation. When he returned to Britain the editors of the medical journals rejected his contributions out of hand. 'They will not admit,' he wrote to a colleague, 'or permit you even to hear of, such indisputable facts, through fear of the consequences' – the consequences being the disapproval of the medical Establishment, which refused to believe that mesmerism was anything more than an illusion, or, more probably, a fraud.

So when anaesthesia finally came, it was via the Davy rather than the Esdaile route. The credit for its re-discovery remains in dispute. There were a number of contenders each mustering some support. In strict chronology, Crawford Long had the best claim. During the early 1840s it became fashionable for groups of young men to get together to inhale nitrous oxide for convivial purposes, much as they might go on a 'pub crawl' today. Long, finding that ether produced the same effect, introduced it as an alternative tipple to his circle of friends in Jefferson, Georgia.

On numerous occasions I inhaled the ether for its exhilarating qualities, and would frequently at some short time discover bruises or painful spots on my person which I had no recollection of causing, and which I felt satisfied were received while under the influence of ether. I noticed my friends while etherised received falls and blows, which I believed sufficient to cause pain on a person not in a state of anaesthesia; and on questioning they uniformly assured me that they did not feel the least pain from these accidents.

Observing these facts I was led to believe that anaesthesia was produced by the inhalation of ether, and that its use would be applicable in surgical operations.

The belief was put to the test on a neighbour from Cobb County, who wanted a tumour removed from the back of his neck; Long operated on him successfully in 1842, ether being administered on a towel. 'The patient continued to inhale ether during the time of the operation, and seemed incredulous until the tumour was shown to him. He gave no evidence of pain during the operation and assured me after it was over that he did not experience the least degree of pain.'

Possibly from fear of censure, Long did not immediately publish an account of his discovery; and it happened that others had had the same idea. Horace Wells, a dentist from Hartford, Conn., began to use nitrous oxide in dental operations, and a demonstration of his technique was staged in Massachusetts General Hospital. Unluckily for Wells, it was not a success; the patient yelled in pain. But a former partner of his, William Morton, persisted with the idea; a further demonstration was arranged in 1846; and John Colling Warren and a board of other eminent Massachusetts surgeons assembled to test 'the *astonishing* claim'. Their scepticism, to judge by an eyewitness account, could almost be felt; and when Morton failed to arrive on time, Warren's contemptuous, 'I presume he is otherwise engaged', caused derisive laughter. But just as the operation was about to be undertaken without his assistance, Morton presented himself. The supreme moment (an eyewitness could proudly boast) had arrived:

The heroic bravery of the man who voluntarily placed himself upon the table, a subject for the surgeon's knife, should be recorded; and his name enrolled upon parchment, which should be hung upon the walls of the surgical ampitheatre in which the operation was performed. His name was Gilbert Abbott. The operation was for a congenital tumour on the left side of the neck, extending along the jaw to the maxillary gland and into the mouth, embracing the margin of the tongue. The operation was successful; and when the patient recovered he declared he had suffered no pain. Dr Warren turned to those present and said, 'Gentlemen, this is no humbug.'

From that moment, the reputation of anaesthetics spread rapidly; and doctors who remained sceptical risked losing their patients. But it was only the beginning of a rancorous dispute about the title of discoverer – and for the patents. The three main contenders were joined by the chemist Charles Jackson, who said that he had suggested the use of ether to Morton; and although this hardly gave him much of a claim to the title, even if it were true, Jackson (who was also to boast that he had suggested the electric tele-graph to Morse) proved a redoubtable and effective fighter.

The melancholy consequence was that none of the four secured the credit to which each felt entitled. Wells went out of his mind with excess of indignation (and inhalation), and committed suicide; Morton tried to do so after a nervous breakdown, and died soon after; and Jackson spent his declining years in a mental hospital. As for Long, though he outlived the others, he never acquired the recognition or respect he craved.

In retrospect, the quarrel seems unnecessary. New ideas and inventions are often discovered independently, and the establishment of precise priorities, though a fascinating academic exercise, is of little value. What is more to the point is the way in which dentists were so intimately concerned. The reason, Richard Shryock suggested in his *Development of Modern Medicine*, is that in those days surgeons were 'oncers'. They did not expect to see a patient twice, and consequently were not unduly worried at causing him unnecessary pain. But a dentist who wanted to attract and keep patients had a strong induce-ment to make his work as painless as possible.

Surgeons, though, realised its significance for them as soon as anaesthesia had established itself – helped by chloroform, which had been discovered in 1828, and turned out to be more effective, though less safe, than ether and nitrous oxide. As anaesthetists have often pointed out, it is chiefly owing to their efforts, with new anaesthetics, general and local, and analgesics, and new techniques of using them, that surgery was enabled to make its most spec-tacular advances. The surgeon, they are inclined to complain, has hogged most of the credit that should rightly be given to them.

There is some truth in this; but anaesthesia has to share the credit with asepsis, without which no decisive advance in surgery would have been possible.

The story of the delays in introducing asepsis is almost as baffling, and as disturbing, as anaesthesia's. At least when anaesthetics had been successfully demonstrated, resistance rapidly crumbled; the few traditionalist objections that remained, such as to its use in childbirth, were religious rather than clinical. Demonstrations of the vital importance of aseptic procedures, though admittedly less dramatic, were to be just as convincing; yet because they went against old customs and prejudices, and because patients did not grasp their significance, the introduction of aseptic procedures was resisted by the very men who should have the best opportunity to observe its value: the surgeons.

As with anaesthesia, this was not for lack of historical evidence. Surgery had first acquired respectability in India in the fourth millennium BC: and although the records of that achievement are scanty, they reveal the emphasis that had been put on strict cleanliness, with regulations about washing hands and cleaning nails – even speaking was prohibited during an operation, for fear the bystander's breath might contaminate the wound. Cleanliness had also been a preoccupation, sometimes a fetish, of the physicians of Babylon and Egypt: and the risk of infection being spread by doctors was referred to in Persian medical literature of the tenth century AD. In Europe Henri de Mondeville insisted:

needles are to be clean, or they will *infect* the wound.

when your dressings have been carefully made, do not interfere with them for some days; keep the air out, for a wound left in contact with the air will suppurate.

With the Renaissance, there was even a tendency for surgeons to become frenetic about the precautions necessary to prevent infection. Avicenna had recommended cautery in place of the knife, if possible, because there was less risk of infection; army surgeons, particularly, were inclined to take him literally – to the disgust of Paracelsus, who insisted that 'in wounds nature is the real physician; all that is necessary is to prevent infection'.

But gradually, realisation of the need for cleanliness in assisting nature disappeared. When the poor were crowded into hospitals, bringing their dirt with them, a punctilious regard for cleanliness at the operating table must have seemed pedantic, and a little ridiculous. In time, some surgeons developed a studied contempt for it. They did not bother to change their clothes, or even to wear an overall for operations – as if to boast to their students that they were not likely to make the kind of mistake that would lead to a spattering of blood or pus. Others used an operating gown, but deliberately kept it unwashed, feeling the same kind of pride in it that people sometimes have for aged scruffy passports, as a measure of past achievement. A stock medical student joke became that so-and-so's operating gown did not have to be hung up at the end of the day; so much blood had caked on it that it stood up on its own.

The surgeon usually credited with being the first to break these habits – or at least the first to do so effectively, in that others were persuaded to follow his example – was Joseph Lister, a London wine merchant's son who had become a surgeon but had retained an interest in bacteriology, because of its importance to his father's trade. When Lister read about Pasteur's work on bacteria and their presence in the air he immediately associated them with the infection he had so often encountered in surgery; and in the 1860s he developed an antiseptic system – taking scrupulous care to give the initial credit to Pasteur in a letter: 'allow me to take this opportunity to tender you my most cordial thanks for having, by your brilliant researches, demonstrated to me the truth of the germ theory of medicine, and thus furnished me with the principle upon which alone the antiseptic system can be carried out.'

Lister's method was to use a spray of carbolic acid, chosen because he had been greatly impressed by a report of its effects on the sewage of the town of Carlisle; 'the admixture of a very small proportion not only preventing all odour from the lands irrigated with the refuse material, but, as it was stated, destroying the entozoa which usually infest cattle fed upon such pastures'. It also, he was pleased to find, exercised a sedative influence on the sensory nerves; rendering it almost painless even on raw flesh. When mixed with blood, too, it hardened into a crust, preventing germs from entering the wound. But the method, although a decided improvement on the earlier procedure, went too far to the other extreme. It was not really necessary, later experimenters found, to try to massacre all the microbes in the vicinity: all that was required was that precautions should be taken by doctors and nurses not to add to the patients' problems by importing them unnecessarily. This was the view which Pasteur eventually expressed to the Academy of Medicine.

This water, this sponge, this lint, with which you wash or cover a wound, deposit germs which have the power of multiplying rapidly within the tissues and which would invariably cause the death of the patient in a very short time, if the vital processes of the body did not counteract them. But alas, the vital resistance is too often impotent; too often the constitution of the wounded, his weakness, his morale, and the inadequate dressing of the wound, oppose an insufficient barrier to the invasion of these infinitely small organisms that, unwittingly, you have introduced into the injured part. If I had the honour of being a surgeon, impressed as I am with the dangers to which the patient is exposed by the microbes present over the surface of all objects, particularly in hospitals, not only would I use none but perfectly clean instruments, but after having cleansed my hands with the greatest care, and subjected them to a rapid flaming, which would expose them to no more inconvenience than that felt by a smoker who passes a glowing coal from one hand to the other, I would use only lint, bandages and sponges previously exposed to a temperature of 130° to 150° C.

Soon, surgeons such as Ernst von Bergmann of Berlin and Lawson Tait of Birmingham, pioneers of abdominal surgery, rejected antisepsis in favour of the strictest possible cleanliness that soap and steam could provide; and out of their experience the aseptic principle developed which, with refinements, was to supersede Lister's antisepsis. But the main opposition to Lister, which was still not entirely routed when he died shortly before the First World War, was from the old guard of surgeons who simply refused to believe there was any need to wash, or to wear clean gowns, and who did their best to make their students feel that Listerism was a ridiculous affectation.

How destructive this professional obduracy could be is best illustrated in the melancholy story of the career of Ignaz Semmelweiss, a Viennese obstetrician who reached the conclusion that puerperal, or child-bed, fever was an act not of God ('the curse of Eve') but of doctors, because they frequently went on their rounds from mothers suffering from the fever, to mothers newly arrived in the lying-in wards, who would catch it as a result. The mortality rate in such wards was sometimes as high as one in four.

Again, the idea that contagion was responsible was not original. It had been put forward by a few eighteenth-century obstetricians and later, forcibly, by Oliver Wendell Holmes.

A physician holding himself in readiness to attend cases of midwifery should never take any active part in the post-mortem examination of cases of puerperal fever . . . If a physician is present at such autopsies, he should use thorough ablution, change every article of dress, and allow twenty-four hours or more to elapse before attending to any case of midwifery . . . On the occurrence of a single case of puerperal fever in his practice, the physician is bound to consider the next female he attends in labour, unless several weeks at least have elapsed, as in danger of being infected by him, and it is his duty to take every precaution to diminish her risk of disease and death. If within a short period, two cases of puerperal fever happen close to each other, in the practice of the same physician . . . he would do wisely to relinquish his obstetrical practice for at least one month . . . The occurrence of three or more closely connected cases, in the practice of one individual . . . is *prima facie* evidence that he is the vehicle of contagion. The physician should make *proper inquiries* concerning nurses and other assistants and give them *timely warning of every suspected source of danger.*

Mental Health

Bedlam, the notorious London asylum; from the final scene of Hogarth's *The Rake's Progress*

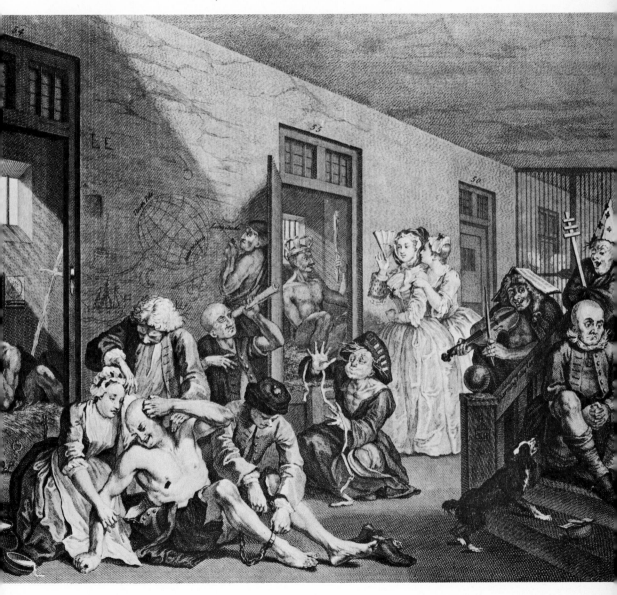

An American naval officer,
William Norris, who was kept
chained up in Bedlam for nine
years, unable to stretch out

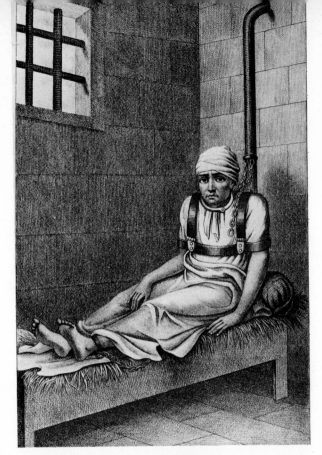

A form of straitjacket in use in a
Paris asylum about 1830, to prevent
a violent patient from injuring
himself

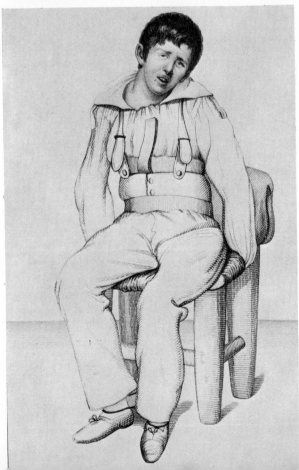

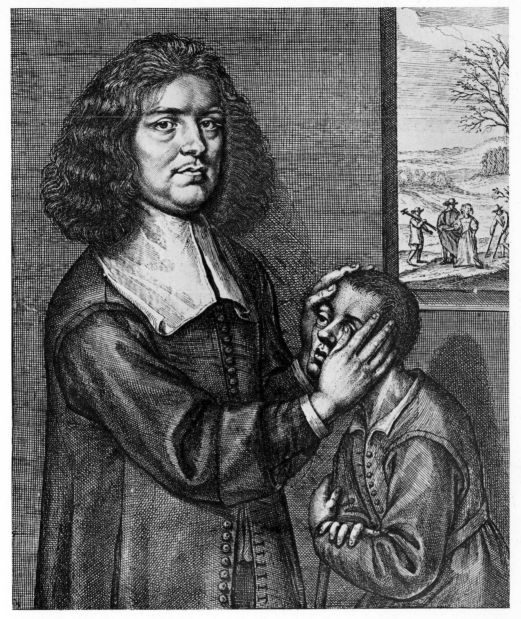

Valentine Greatraks the Irishman, an exponent of magnetic cures in the mid seventeenth century

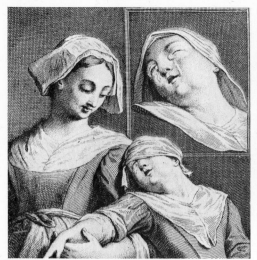
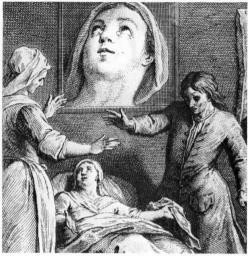

Marie Carteri who had suffered from an eye ailment: before and after her miraculous cure at the tomb of the Jansenist saint, Blessed François de Paris (d. 1727)

Crowds of sufferers at the tomb of François de Paris about 1735, hoping for miraculous cures for their ailments

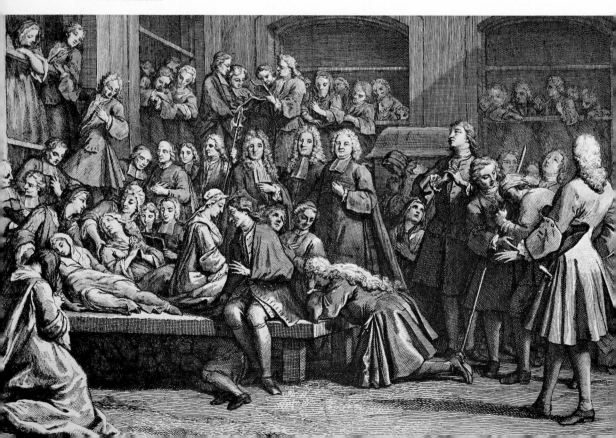

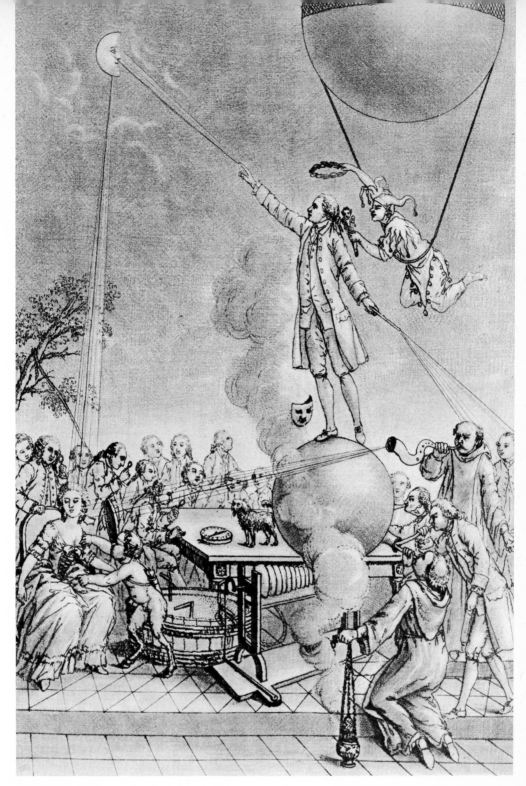

'Burlesque Apotheosis' of Mesmer, the originator of animal magnetism, showing the bath, and other paraphernalia used at his sessions

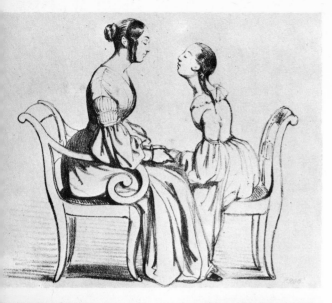

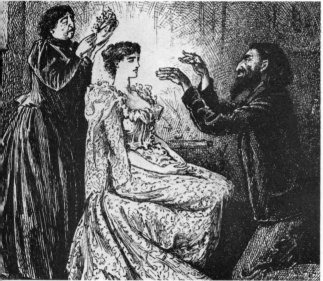

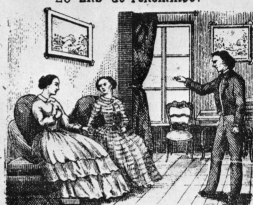

Above left: Anna M. mesmerizing her younger sister, while herself in a mesmeric trance. From a medical account of *Facts in Mesmerism* (1840)

Below left: Svengali in Du Maurier's *Trilby* exemplified the popular image of the mesmerist

Right: Advertisement for fashionable sessions of magnetism and somnambulism in Paris in the mid nineteenth century

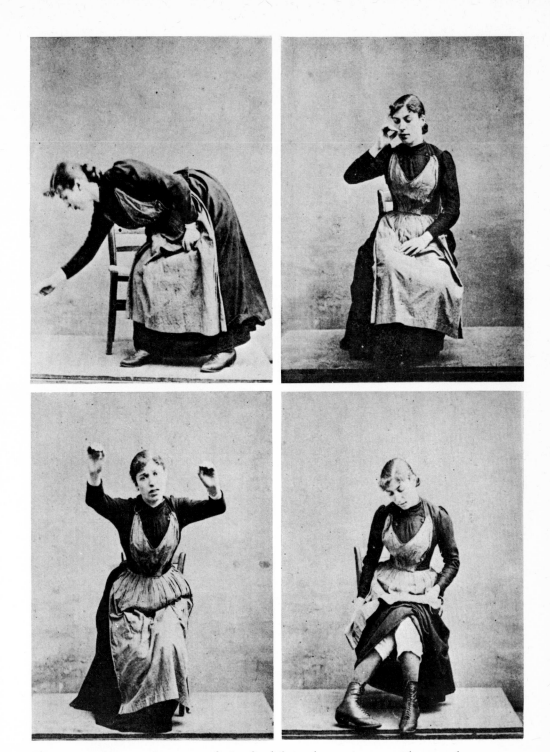

Woman reacting to various external stimuli while in a hypnotic trance. Photographs illustrating an experiment by Jean Charcot

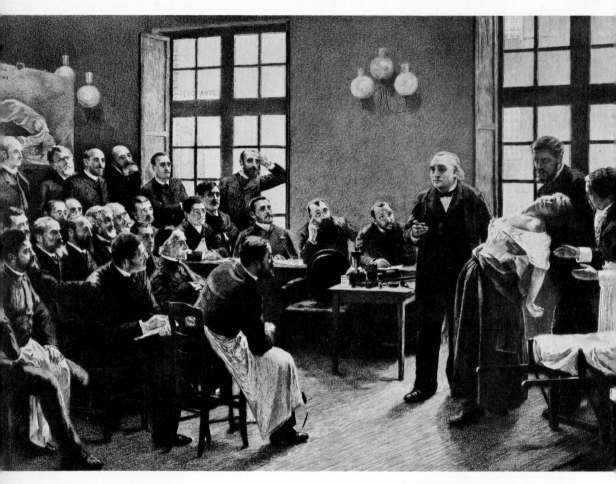

Charcot lecturing at the Salpêtrière, a print which Freud had above his desk in Vienna

One of Charcot's patients, suffering from persecution mania, in the metal 'armour' which he made to protect himself

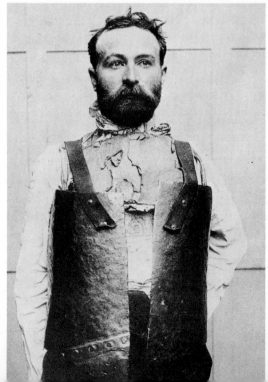

Holmes read his paper on the contagiousness of medical fever to a Boston audience in 1843 – at the time that Wells, not far away, was making his experiments with anaesthetics. Holmes confessed that he was not certain how the contagion was spread, 'whether it be by the atmosphere the physician carries about him into the sick chamber, or by the direct application of the virus to the absorbing surfaces with which his hand comes into contact'; and he conceded that there might be other causes besides contagion – like small-pox, its incidence waxed and waned unaccountably. But he was prepared to state dogmatically that the disease was 'so far contagious as to be frequently carried from patient to patient by physicians and nurses'; so that if it were shown that lives were being sacrificed to ignorance or blindness, 'the common instincts of humanity will silence every attempt to explain away their responsibility'.

Holmes' obstetric colleagues hardly even bothered to be angry with him; they simply ignored the evidence he had produced, and dismissed his virus contagion idea as airy nonsense. One of them announced that he preferred to attribute puerperal fever cases 'to accident, or Providence, of which I can form a conception, rather than to a contagion of which I cannot form any idea, at least as to this particular malady'. And – this being before Pasteur's microbiological discoveries – his complacency was shared by most of his colleagues.

Semmelweiss does not appear to have been aware of Holmes' existence: he came to hold the contagion theory from personal experience. As the story runs, he found an expectant mother in a waiting-room crying because, she said, she had been assigned to the students' ward, rather than to the mid-wives'; and this had come to be regarded as a death sentence. Then in 1847 one of his friends died after injuring himself at a post-mortem; the symptoms, Semmelweiss noticed, were similar to those of women who had died of puerperal sepsis, suggesting to him that the reason mortality was high in the student's wards was not because they were incompetent but because they attended post mortems; midwives did not. Semmelweiss tested the theory by ordering the students to wash their hands thoroughly in a disinfectant solution between each case they attended; the death rate from puerperal sepsis in their wards immediately dropped to one in a hundred. Puerperal fever, Semmel-weiss could confidently announce, was nothing more than induced blood-poisoning; and therefore relatively easy to banish.

Semmelweiss did not spare himself:

The variations in the mortality as they occurred in the divisions can be attributed to the special occupations of the various members of the staff. As an assistant I took special interest in pathological anatomy. I dissected endlessly to discover why these women were dying. The mortality soared. Consequently must I here make my confession that God only knows the numbers of women whom I have consigned prematurely to the grave. I have occupied myself with the cadaver to an extent reached by few obstetricians. However painful and depressing the recognition may be, there is no advantage in concealment; if the misfortune is not to remain permanent, the truth must be brought home to all concerned . . .

But some concerned would not listen to the truth. Of the countless instances of professional blindness when confronted with a reasonable hypothesis backed by convincing evidence, the opposition to Semmelweiss is the most saddening. He happened to produce his theory at the worst possible time – when professional complacency was still entrenched, before Pasteur's work was known. And Semmelweiss was not prepared to obey the conventions of polite medical disputation. Holmes had said that though there was 'deadly incompatibility and exterminating warfare between doctrines', there was no quarrel between men. Semmelweiss bluntly called his opponents 'murderers'; and they retaliated by getting him dismissed from his post. He obtained another, at Budapest, where he wrote his work *The Cause, Concept and Prophylaxis of Puerperal Fever*. Still he found himself derided. Holmes, in later life, could indulge himself with the quiet boast: 'Others had cried out against the terrible evil before I did, but I think I shrieked my warning louder and longer than any of them – before the little army of microbes was marched in to support my position.' But Semmelweiss did not live to see his theory finally vindicated. Whether the insanity which overtook him was caused, as some believed, by the strain of violent controversy, and by brooding on the wrong done to him by colleagues, has been disputed; but nobody is likely to dispute Garrison's summing-up: 'he is one of medicine's martyrs and, in the future, will be one of its far-shining names, for every child-bearing woman owes something to him.'

The impetus that anaesthesia and asepsis gave to surgery was immense; and from that time on operations which had previously been impracticable became relatively easy – brain operations, lung operations and stomach operations; operations for the removal of diseased appendages; operations simply to discover if it was necessary to operate. Yet when the wonders of modern medicine are spoken of, it is not normally the achievements of surgery that are being recalled. The advance that comes first to mind was in microbiology – linked with the name of its progenitor, Louis Pasteur.

Microbiology: Pasteur

That diseases were spread by invisible organisms had often been propounded, even as far back as Roman times, by men who were seeking to explain the reasons for epidemics; but as the means to prove it were lacking, the thesis tended to be ignored. Then, in the sixteenth century Fracastoro had put forward his theory, which came just about as close to the truth as was possible in the circumstances of his time, dividing infectious diseases into three categories: direct contagion through touch; indirect contagion through, say, sleeping in the same sheets that an infected man had slept in; and airborne transmission on the same basis as pollen – the disease agents, Fracastoro believed, being too small to be visible by the naked eye. And two centuries later Marcus Plenciz of Vienna had argued convincingly that disease must be caused by living micro-organisms.

The ground, then, had been prepared for Pasteur; and even some of the discoveries which are ordinarily thought of as his had been made earlier by others: Agostino Bassi of Lodi, who had shown that the silkworm disease was caused by a parasitic fungus, and how it could be controlled, had published his findings in 1836. Nevertheless, there is justice in their yielding of pride of place to Pasteur, because it was his intuitions, backed by meticulous research, that transformed microbiology from a jumble of disconnected ideas into a system, and showed how it could be exploited for the benefit of the human race.

Of the two contributions to medicine on which Pasteur's fame rests, the most influential was connected with specific microbes. Again, he was not the first to make the discovery – but he was the first to demonstrate it convincingly and once he had shown the way, the identification of the various microbes and viruses became relatively simple.

Inevitably, Pasteur had to fight so strenuously to establish this connection, against traditionalists who simply refused to believe that micro-organisms could be responsible for disease, that in the process his name became identified with an unduly narrow interpretation of his findings. He himself continually reiterated that he had not proved that microbes were the cause of disease: they might simply be the agents. Even when he showed that it was the anthrax bacillus itself, and not its toxic properties disseminated in the surrounding fluid, which was destructive, he nevertheless insisted that the bacillus might not be directly responsible; it might, say, produce a virus, as yet undiscovered, which did the damage. And this qualification was not simply academic. For the purposes of controlling disease, he realised it might be necessary to think in terms not of slaughtering the bacillus, but of finding out why it should disseminate dangerous viruses; in order to find ways of disarming it, and making its presence less of a danger to humans.

The importance of this reservation was to be emphasised later when research workers were disconcerted to find what they had been taught to regard was *the* cause of a disease leading an apparently harmless existence in 'carriers' – men and women who were found to be hosts to the virus identified with a disease, but did not suffer from the symptoms. This suggested that the cause of disease must sometimes be not the virus, but the 'terrain' it encountered: in certain circumstances individuals, or groups, must have some way of coming to terms with potentially hostile disease agents and disarming them. This had been Claude Bernard's view; and it was vigorously propounded by the German Max von Pettenkofer, also a chemist, but deeply impressed with the importance of the terrain.

Pettenkofer's views did not at first bring him into conflict with the microbiologists because his recommendations were often the same as their's would have been. He insisted upon, and obtained, clean water for Munich from the snow-capped mountains nearby because it was aesthetically satisfying and because it tasted good – rather than because it was germ-free; but it brought down the Munich typhoid mortality figures by 75 per cent. Diseases, he was prepared (though reluctantly) to admit, *might* have a specific virus attached, but the virus was not the cause: it could only work where there was a disease proneness, owing to bad constitutional or environmental circumstances. To prove his point he acquired from Ludwig Koch in 1892 what in ordinary circumstances was regarded as a lethal dose of the cholera virus, which he drank with no adverse effects other than mild diarrhoea; and members of his staff, emboldened, also took the dose and were unharmed by it.

This would in no way have disconcerted Pasteur, aware as he was of the

156

limitations of an exclusively microbiological interpretation of the cause of disease; on his deathbed he insisted that Claude Bernard had been right about the terrain's importance vis-à-vis the germ. But many of his followers ignored this qualification. The theory that germs were the cause of disease had a simplicity about it that was extremely attractive for research workers: it brought medicine into the confines of the laboratory. By breeding viruses – in test tubes, if possible – and experimenting with them on animals, the secrets of diseases could be explored, and their cures developed, without reference to the outside world, at least until the time came to try them on volunteers. The notion of the influence of the terrain, by contrast, was complex, embracing not only body but mind – perhaps even soul, though souls by this time were rarely taken into account. To the mechanistically minded, the germ theory was much more attractive.

For Pasteur, the contest between the germ and the terrain school was in any case to some extent irrelevant; because the therapeutic method – his second great contribution – which he developed was capable of satisfying the requirements of both. Essentially, it was a revival of inoculation – but with this difference: that the immunising dose was controlled. Pasteur hit upon a way of achieving this by accident. In 1879, he had begun to experiment with inducing cholera into chickens; and one batch of cholera germs that had been kept for a few months during the summer failed to kill. More important, when the chickens who had survived were injected with a fresh and ordinarily fatal dose, they survived. At once, Pasteur recognised the analogy with Jenner's cow girl: and he adopted the term vaccination to describe the method which was soon to save so many lives in a variety of diseases: introducing the agents of a disease in a weakened condition into a healthy patient, whose defences deal with them, giving him immunity to the disease in the process.

Pasteur's vaccination was quickly shown to be effective on animals; with human beings he was understandably more cautious, and there is still some doubt whether the best known of his triumphs, his rabies' treatment, was really as efficacious as it seemed to be (as few people who are bitten by mad dogs develop rabies, it is difficult to make a trustworthy assessment). But other researchers left no doubt that he had been on the right track. His work was followed up by an exile from Russia who came to work at his Paris institute: Elie Metchnikoff, who translated the life force from an abstraction into bio-chemical terms. Watching cells' behaviour under a microscope, the inspiration came to him that this was how the body's defence forces worked; and experiment revealed that the white blood corpuscles, or phagocytes, move into action whenever an invasion of viruses or other potentially injurious agents is reported. This, then, was the explanation why the Turkish crones' smallpox remedy had worked: in dealing with the attenuated viruses, the phagocytes gained the requisite experience to deal with a later attack of smallpox even if, when it came, it was on a much more massive scale.

Why, then, should vaccination not be the answer to all germ- or virus-borne diseases? For a time, this approach looked extremely promising. Von Behring, a Prussian army surgeon, showed in 1890 that attenuated serum from animals immunised them against diphtheria, and could be used to give human beings immunity. Theobald Smith of Harvard discovered that it was not always necessary to inoculate with attenuated viruses; in certain cases, dead ones would do. In London, Almroth Wright perfected an anti-typhoid injection; and other immunisation procedures followed – as army recruits and immigrants were to find, sometimes painfully.

But there were setbacks; notably in connection with TB, where Robert Koch's work ended in failure. Koch had actually been the first, in 1876, to show beyond possibility of doubt that an infectious disease – anthrax – was related to specific micro-organisms; before even Pasteur. Soon, the agents of gonor-rhea, of typhoid, of malaria and other diseases were isolated by researchers; but what appeared to be the most resounding triumph was reserved for Koch when, in 1882, he was able to report that he had discovered the tubercle bacillus – thereby finally disposing of the belief that TB was a nutritional (or an emotional) disorder. And the following year, with his discovery of the cholera vibrio, it seemed that he was destined to surpass even Pasteur.

For Koch, it was not sufficient to find the culprits. He wanted to be able to exterminate them; the work of his assistant, von Behring, on diphtheria gave him the necessary lead; and in 1891, he announced that he had discovered the cure for TB: tuberculin, made from attenuated bacilli. The impact of the news was enormous; from all over the world, TB sufferers set out for Berlin in the hope that tuberculin would save them. For a time, expectations remained high that it was indeed the cure; but they were dashed by adverse reports, and gradually realisation grew that it was a failure. Evidently there must be some disorders, such as diphtheria, against which it was relatively easy to provide immunity; others, such as TB, where the difficulties were more formidable. They have continued insuperable to this day, in spite of continual research.

Why one disease should respond to immunisation and not another remains unexplained; but it was to come as a relief when polio was found to be one which *did* respond. Striking though the public reaction to Koch's tuberculin had been, it was puny compared to the emotional wave which spread over America and many other parts of the world when it was announced, with all the publicity an experienced PR machine could provide, that Jonas Salk had found a polio vaccine. It had struck indiscriminately at the children of rich and poor alike, and left its mark on many into adulthood: it had aroused the same fears as smallpox, and its conquest seemed a miracle. As the months passed, some of the initial enthusiasm began to wane. Doctors pointed out that at its worst, polio was not all that serious a scourge in terms of numbers affected (Louis Lasagna sardonically has noted that more people die from anaesthetic complications during surgery each year than from polio). Besides, its incidence had begun to decline before the vaccine came on the market – from nearly 40 cases per 100,000 of the population in 1942, to 15 in 1952: so there was some doubt whether the Salk vaccine had been responsible for the further decline. But at least polio had been reduced, whatever the reasons, to negligible proportions.

Other disorders, such as influenza, proved intractable: the reason being, it is now supposed, that any of a hundred or more different viruses can be identified as disease agents, and it is not possible to give an immunising injection of all of them. There was also the risk to some people of what came to be called anaphylactic shock. Unharmed by the initial injection, a few patients would react violently to a second one; the phagocytes seemed to have been all too well prepared, and their reaction to the interloper too violent for the body's safety – as when armed police, firing at criminals, hit innocent bystanders. Again, Sydenham's hypothesis was vindicated: the violent symptoms were caused not by a disease agent, but the body's efforts – in this case, misguided – to fight one off. And these false reactions, it gradually came to be recognised, could be held responsible for a wide range of disorders, where individuals were allergic or hypersensitive. Asthma, for example, could most easily be explained as a consequence of the life force coming into operation by sending supplies of fluid to clear the nasal passages, and to sweep out an obstruction, even though the obstruction – as it might be pollen – was harmless.

159

Immunisation could be extremely costly, if carried out comprehensively; it also met with conscientious objections, and sometimes apathy. The possibility that there might be an easier alternative method occurred to Paul Ehrlich, working in Berlin. Von Behring's discovery of anti-toxins, he was later to write, had opened up a new vista in pharmacology and therapeutics; 'for anti-toxins and antibacterial substances are, as it were, magic bullets which strike only those objects for whose destruction they have been produced by the organism'. Suppose, then, that research could discover bullets which would do the body's work for it, by knocking out the virus direct? Ehrlich went to work to experiment with arsenical compounds. It was trial and error: but in 1910 the 606th trial produced Salvarsan, the first of the 'wonder drugs', hailed as a specific against syphilis, and earning Ehrlich the title – from Victor Robinson – of a saviour of the race; 'as a therapeutic achievement, the production of salvarsan (606) and neo-salvarsan (914) had never been surpassed'.

The fact that a 'neo-salvarsan' proved necessary, though, was significant. The original drug proved less efficacious than was at first believed; and for a while no successor appeared to perform the same functions in other disorders. Then, in the 1920s, hope was renewed when two Toronto doctors, Frederick Banting and Charles Best, found Insulin; and when a few years later the value was discovered of liver extract in treating patients with pernicious anemia. Meanwhile, too, the diagnosis of disease had been improving, not only with the help of the microscope, but by Röntgen's discovery in 1895 of X-rays, which simplified the detection of many internal disorders – so much so that it could be assumed the stethoscope would soon follow the carafe out of fashion as a medical symbol.

But improvements in diagnosis were of little help unless followed by improvements in treatment; and these lagged until in 1935, Gerhard Domagk revealed that a dye, prontosil red, gave protection to mice against streptococci. Both Koch and Ehrlich had followed up the clue, discovered earlier, that some dyes had a microbiological action – Ehrlich had hoped they would provide him with his magic bullets. Now, the sulfa drugs developed from prontosil red turned out to be effective not only against individual disorders: they were used with success against meningitis, VD, and many other infections, as well as against streptococci.

For anybody under fifty it is not easy to grasp what a difference this made.

Dostoevsky summed up the situation at the end of the nineteenth century, through the mouth of Ivan Karamazov's doppelganger:

I've consulted all sorts of doctors; they can diagnose excellently, they will tell you all your symptoms, they have your illness at their finger tips, but they've no idea how to cure you. I happened to come across a very enthusiastic medical student. 'You may die,' he told me, 'but at least you'll have a very good idea of what illness you are dying of.'

And as late as the 1920s, the Professor of Applied Pharmacology at Harvard, H. W. Haggard, had to admit that medicine could 'do little to repair damage from diseases. Except in a few cases, medicine cannot cure. It can only support the strength and lessen the pain for sufferers, and at best it keeps him alive until nature heals him.' Nobody knew why meningitis or pneumonia struck; and when they did, there was little to be done but wait and hope. The new drugs, particularly the antibiotics, offered the prospect of a life free from such hazards. With intensive research, and a little luck, the fear of disease could be banished. A few days in hospital, a short convalescence, and the victim would be back as healthy as before – perhaps all the better for the rest.

The prospect was not to be fulfilled. The sulfa drugs saved thousands of patients who would otherwise have died, and cleared up tens of thousands of apparently intractable infections. But ugly side-effects began to present themselves, with some fatalities. So the news that an even more effective and safer drug had been found – penicillin, the first of the antibiotics – was greeted with relief. Penicillin, it was claimed, could achieve even more than the sulfa drugs had done, more safely and more expeditiously.

So it could, and did; but gradually, cases of what were regarded as hypersensitivity to it began to be reported; along with frequent minor side-effects such as rashes and skin lesions. Even more disconcertingly there developed, in a depressingly short time, bacterial strains resistant to the drug. Evidently the evolutionary mechanism had been at work. Destructive though penicillin had been, its killing power had been far from complete; and the organisms which survived were immunised as if by inoculation. Some grew more virulent. Pasteur had warned that epidemics may arise because micro-organisms which have been giving no trouble can suddenly be roused, and turn vicious; antibiotics appeared sometimes to act as irritants. In the late

1940s and early 1950s new antibiotics were brought out which the makers claimed were even more effective than the old, and could deal with the resistant strains; but some of them turned out to be more dangerous than penicillin. The toll from side-effects began to reach disturbing proportions.

Iatrogenic illness – as disorders arising out of medical treatment, other than those arising from accidents, have come to be called – must have been a frequent occurrence in the days of polypharmacy; but its existence was rarely noted, as, if the patient died from treatment it was assumed he died from the disease. With antibiotics the symptoms were too consistent: it was no longer possible to escape the conclusion that they resulted from the administration of the drug. By the 1950s the literature of side-effects attributable to antibiotics, and to other new drugs, was voluminous, and by the 1960s iatrogenic illness had become one of the most widespread and serious of the medical profession's problems.

It was not only the antibiotics which produced unwanted symptoms. After the Second World War the pharmaceutical industry entered into a period of massive expansion, during which hundreds of new drugs poured onto the market every year. Some of them were variations of established drugs, like insulin or penicillin; but many broke new ground – the most striking of them being cortisone.

Like insulin, cortisone was related to the work of Bernard and others who in the nineteenth century had re-introduced a form of humoralism, relating the body's disorders to the malfunction of glands. The hormone cortisone was isolated in the Mayo Clinic in the 1930s, and used clinically after the war, initially for rheumatoid arthritis, with spectacular success. 'If the word "miraculous" may ever be used in referring to the effects of a remedy', Lord Horder claimed, 'it could surely be excused here.' Cripples long bed-ridden were able to get up and walk; arthritics lost the stiffness and the pain in their limbs.

The side-effects, though, turned out to be disturbing. Women's faces ballooned, or grew hirsute: ugly skin disorders were reported; heart disease, stomach ulcers and insanity occasionally followed cortisone treatment, and it left patients highly susceptible to certain infectious disorders. Clearly, playing around with hormones often disturbed the body's homeostatic balance: a result that was also to follow treatment with other drugs, including later refinements of cortisone. Often new drugs saved lives and relieved suffering;

but their over-all results were not impressive, when their failures and the damage they sometimes did (not to mention their cost) were set off against them. And few of them actually cured patients; usually they brought only temporary relief.

The antibiotics frequently cured; but as their use bred resistant strains of microbes, they quickly became obsolescent, requiring new antibiotics to replace them – or mixtures of antibiotics, used in the hope that one of the components, at least, would be effective. Once the idea was established, elaborations followed: mixtures of different types of drug, particularly if one was a tranquilliser, could be held to have excellent therapeutic possibilities. So doctors' treatment, instead of taking heed of chemotherapy's risks, tended to become more dependent on drugs – and to some extent on polypharmacy, so long discredited.

This, in spite of the fact that evidence had begun to appear to show that a great deal of drug therapy had been not merely risky, but unnecessary. When the British Medical Research Council compared cortisone with aspirin, to decide which was the drug of choice for patients contracting rheumatoid arthritis, its report concluded that cortisone's introduction had 'not materially affected the prognosis' and that at least in the first few years 'medication with aspirin is more often likely to prove satisfactory than medication with cortisone'. Why, then, had cortisone given to all appearances such remarkable results when it was first introduced?

The reason lay only to a limited extent in the power of the drug itself. The more potent therapeutic force must have been suggestion. It had long been realised that certain people were susceptible to it, and could be 'cured' by the administration of coloured water: the term 'placebo' – from the Latin 'I will please' – had long since established itself to describe any mock drug given for that purpose. But the assumption had been that only the gullible few were taken in – and that they were not really ill: their symptoms were hysterical or functional. But now, the suspicion began to arise that placebo effect must have been very much more pervasive, operating through the enthusiasm of doctors transmitting itself to many of their patients, not just to hypochondriacs. To verify this hypothesis, researchers began to make tests, giving placebo – dummy – pills to some patients, and the real pill to others, and comparing the results. As a refinement, to prevent the doctors' conscious or unconscious bias affecting results, some of these tests were carried out 'double blind' – neither the doctor nor his patients being allowed to know which were getting the pill and which the placebo; the results could then be analysed later by independent assessors.

The results were startling. In 1933 two British researchers, comparing the effectiveness of the drugs then in use for angina pectoris, had found that almost forty per cent of patients gained relief from bicarbonate of soda. The implications of this experiment struck the Harvard researcher, Dr Henry K. Beecher, and he began to investigate the whole subject of placebo reactions. In 1955 the *Journal* of the American Medical Association printed his article, 'The Powerful Placebo', including a list of the results that he and other researchers had achieved. It showed that over a range of common disorders – coughs, colds, headaches, seasickness, anxiety, and pains of various kinds – an average of over a third of all patients were satisfactorily relieved by the administration of a placebo.

This research explained much that had previously been baffling about the results of treatment. It had not been only the gullible who were taken in by quack remedies; provided that the imagination was caught by confidence either in the doctor or the drug, a sizable minority – and in some cases, a majority – of patients were placebo-reactors. No wonder, then, that new drugs had so often given impressive results, only to disappoint later.

To utilise this knowledge in treatment, however, presented obvious difficulties. It could work only so long as the patients did not know that they were receiving placebos; and for the doctor to mislead them about the drug he was prescribing, though it might be justified by results, could eventually lead to a breach in the doctor–patient relationship. In any case, with few exceptions, doctors have remained wedded to chemotherapy, and unwilling to face the implications of the discovery.

Yet those implications are clear. Humanity owes far less to new drugs than has commonly been thought; and those historians of medicine who, like Shryock, tried to redress the balance by recording the achievements in the public health sector, have been unfairly neglected. At the height of penicillin's fame, a warning came from J. P. Lockhart Mummery in his *Nothing New Under the Sun*: 'We can have no hope', he wrote, 'of evolving an immunity by natural process to bacterial and virus diseases since, even if it were possible for man to evolve immunity to virus disease, these parasites could evolve a new variety much more rapidly than any immunity man can evolve to resist their invasion.' The Berlin thoracic surgeon, Ernst Sauerbruch, had earlier expressed a fear that the bacteriological concept of disease might have led medical science into a blind alley. And it is now possible to see that the decisive advances in the control of infectious diseases were achieved not by slaying viruses and microbes, but – as Pettenkofer did – preventing them from making nuisances of themselves: improving water supplies to eliminate cholera and typhoid; systematic de-lousing to control typhus; draining swamps or making them otherwise mosquito-proof to reduce malaria; and so on. True, these measures sometimes had to be supplemented where such control proved impossible: quinine substitutes and DDT were needed to keep down malaria and typhus when preventive measures were inadequate in the Second World War. And in the case of polio, no preventive measure has been found other than vaccines. Nonetheless, the chief credit for the astonishingly rapid fall in mortality rates from diseases over the past century must be given primarily to the advances in public health, which have enabled civilised communities to enjoy standards of hygiene almost as high as those of the Ancient Romans.

Even Pasteur's biographer, René Dubos – though he did not dispute that microbiology had had considerable value in improving diagnosis, and providing a rational basis for prophylactic and therapeutic procedures – refused to accept the commonly held assumption that the control of infectious diseases dates from the introduction of modern chemotherapy. The introduction of a new drug has often led to a diminution in the destructiveness of a disease, but it can rarely be proved that the drug is responsible. Several diseases, notably scarlet fever and measles, have declined in virulence in the last hundred years for no discernible reason. The decrease in mortality caused by infection, Dubos pointed out, 'began almost a century ago and has continued ever since at a fairly constant rate irrespective of the use of any specific therapy. The effect of anti-bacterial drugs is but a ripple on the wave which has been wearing down the mortality caused by infection in our communities.'

Public Health

Although public health measures had been an integral feature of several earlier civilisations – India, Babylon, Egypt, Rome – they had come to be neglected largely owing to constitutional instability, which made it difficult for governments or civic authorities to pay for or enforce the necessary measures. By the time stability returned, their value had been forgotten.

From time to time individuals urged the need for greater civic efforts – Defoe put forward a plan for a health insurance scheme – but none attracted much attention until in the eighteenth and early nineteenth century Johann Frank introduced Germans to what is recognisably the modern concept of public health services 'from the womb to the tomb'. The first practical reforms on a national scale, however, were taken in Britain. Townsmen had been accustomed to get rid of their refuse, including excreta, into the street; where at night it was collected for sale as manure. As towns grew larger this method became increasingly inefficient and obnoxious, as well as unsafe, and at the end of the eighteenth century Acts of Parliament were passed which authorised civic authorities to construct new paved streets that could be drained and cleaned. The appearance of wide dignified streets, with tall dignified houses, only served to emphasise the contrast with the slums festering behind them; and to Jeremy Bentham and the Utilitarians it was obvious that there was a need for much wider powers to deal with housing, sanitation and health, because the industrial revolution which then taking place was nicely calculated to destroy the health of the workers.

They were compelled to work extremely long hours – a sixteen-hour day was commonplace – in wretched conditions with little light (in Britain a window tax imposed for revenue had led to windows being blocked up, wherever possible), inadequate ventilation and overcrowding. And in addition to the disorders that arise out of such conditions – bronchitis, rheumatism, spinal lesions – occupational diseases began to flourish: silicosis, and 'phossy jaw', poisoning from lead or mercury.

Thomas Southwood Smith, a Scots clergyman, worked with Bentham to draw up a comprehensive code; but acquaintance with the subject forced him to realise that it was not just a matter of ministering to the sick, and educating people to better habits of hygiene. In his own words:

The room of a fever patient, in a small and heated apartment of London, with no perflation of fresh air, is perfectly analogous to a stagnant pool in Ethiopia full of the bodies of dead locusts. The poison generated in both cases is the same; the difference is merely in the degree of its potency. Nature with her burning sun, her stilled and pent-up wind, her stagnant and teeming marsh, manufactures plague on a large and fearful scale. Poverty in her hut, covered with her rags, surrounded by her filth, striving with all her might to keep out the pure air and to increase the heat, imitates nature; the process and the product are the same, the only difference is in the magnitude of the result. Penury and ignorance can thus, at any time and in any place, create a mortal plague.

Southwood Smith's dilemma was neatly summed up in his aphorism about prevalence of hookworm in certain primitive communities. All that was needed to banish the disorder, he pointed out, was shoes; 'but who is to provide the shoes?' It would be much less expensive, he insisted, as well as more effective, to take preventive measures in Britain in the form of better housing, clothing, diet, and so on, rather than allow unhealthy stunted children to grow up into weak and disease-prone adults.

To banish disease, then, it was necessary first to banish penury; and this would require not merely massive expenditure, but also a breach in the ingenious *laissez faire* edifice that had been constructed to justify the methods of the new entrepreneurs. Their attitude to the radical agitator (as they thought of him) who wanted better housing, hygiene and health services, was the same as their attitude to the trade unionist who wanted higher wages, or the philanthropist who campaigned for shorter hours: any impediment to the free market in labour, anything which raised production costs, would destroy the competitiveness of their goods in the world's markets, compel them to reduce output, and perhaps put them out of business – so that the worker would be worse off than before. But against this, there had to be set the risk that bad working and living conditions would create a revolutionary ferment – the Chartist movement in Britain, and Communism on the Continent, gave cause for alarm. There was also the fear that they might spread diseases which would threaten rich as well as poor; and in the 1830s the Whig governments at last began tentatively to grapple with the health problems presented by a rapidly growing population, much of it on the subsistence level, and epidemic-prone.

The most energetic advocate of public health laws was Edwin Chadwick, secretary of the Poor Law Commission and a persistent campaigner for better sanitary measures; his report published in 1850 on *The Sanitary Condition of the Labouring Population of Great Britain* incontrovertibly established the proposition that poverty and sickness were linked, and that it was hopeless to think or eradicating disease except in terms of eradicating poverty.

That the various forms of epidemic, endemic, and other disease caused, or aggravated, or propagated chiefly amongst the labouring classes by atmospheric impurities, produced by decomposing animal and vegetable substances, by damp and filth and close overcrowded dwellings, prevail amongst the population in every part of the kingdom, whether dwelling in separate houses, in rural villages, in small towns, in the larger towns – as they have been found to prevail in the lowest districts of the metropolis . . .

That such disease, wherever its attacks are frequent, is always found in connexion where those circumstances are removed by drainage, proper cleansing, better ventilation and other means of diminishing atmospheric impurity; the frequency and intensity of such disease is abated, and where the removal of the noxious agencies appears to be complete, such disease almost entirely disappears.

The primary and most important measures, and at the same time the most practicable, and within the recognized province of administration, are drainage, the removal of all refuse from habitations, streets and roads, and the improvement of the supplies of water.

This now self-evident proposition horrified the authorities, in spite of the evidence they had just been given by the great famine in Ireland. The famine itself was brought on by a blight attacking the Irish peasants' only means of subsistence, the potato. There was plenty of food available in Ireland, a corn-growing country at the time; but the British government, wedded to *laissez faire*, would not allow it to be distributed, except through the ordinary marketing channels. As the peasants had no money, there were no ordinary marketing channels; and they starved. Epidemics followed, and were soon out of control; it was impossible even to guess what proportion of the million fatalities died of starvation or of disease – public works eventually set up to provide employment and purchasing power being too few and too late. If the authorities could cling to *laissez faire* even in those circumstances, it is not surprising that Chadwick's plans, envisaging as they did a considerable expenditure of public money and interference with private domestic arrangements, should have been rejected. His enemies became more numerous and more influential, and in the 1850s he was given a liberal pension on condition that, as he ruefully commented, he would 'leave dirt and disease alone'. Years after his death, almost all the measures he had recommended had to be introduced piecemeal by later governments.

In the meantime, doctors had to do the best they could in conditions which, to judge from contemporary descriptions, were hardly better than those of

Public Health and Modern Drugs

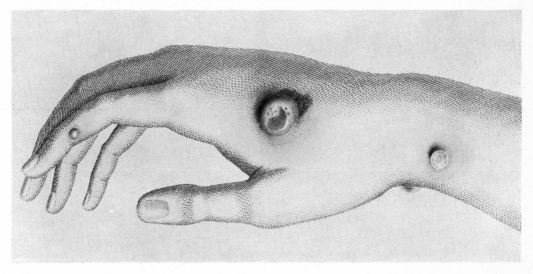

Hand of the milkmaid Sarah Nelmes infected with cowpox, from which Edward Jenner
conceived the idea of vaccination

The Wonderful Effect of the New Inoculation by Gillray, spokesman for the many fierce opponents
of vaccination

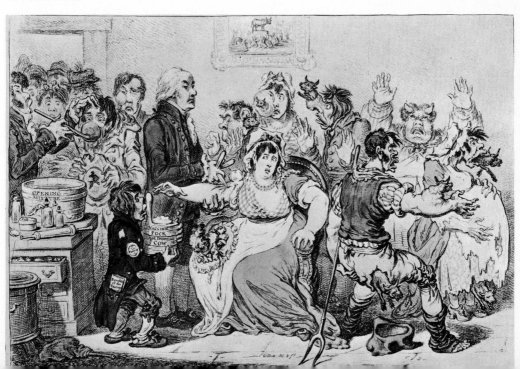

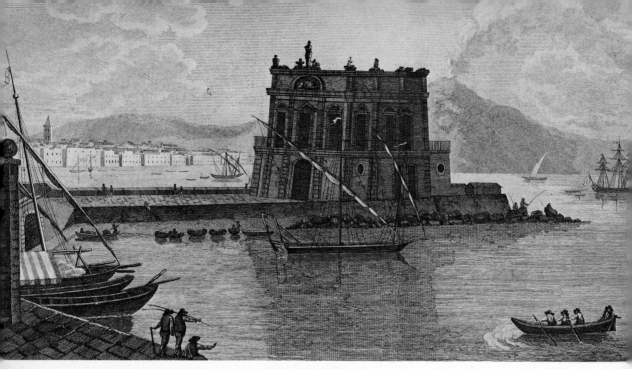

The Health Office at Naples in the eighteenth century, which enforced quarantine regulations to protect the health of the town

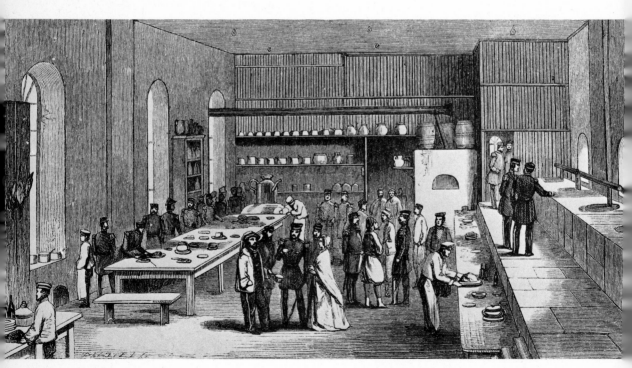

Kitchen at Scutari run by Alexis Soyer, chef of the London Reform Club. Besides working in the Crimea, he opened soup kitchens for the poor during the Irish famine and in the London slums, using cheap raw materials as economically and nourishingly as possible

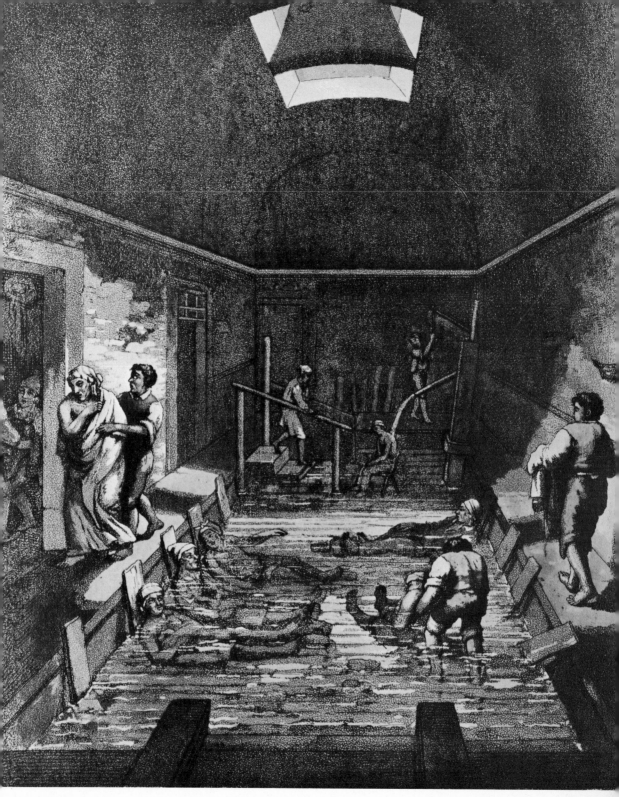

Caldas da Reinha in Portugal, one of the many therapeutic baths which were particularly popular in the nineteenth century.

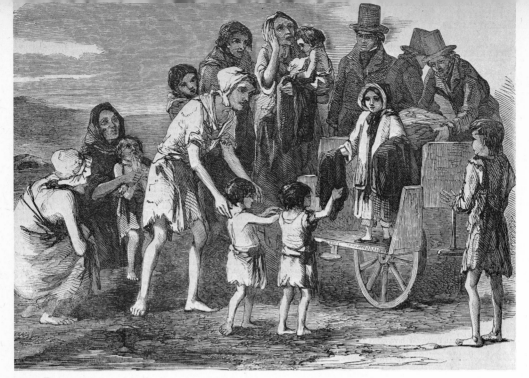

Miss Kennedy distributing clothing at Kilrush during the Irish famine of the 1840s, which produced conditions reminiscent of the famines of the Middle Ages

Plague-spot near the London gas-works, South Lambeth, in 1843, probably caused by contaminated water-supply

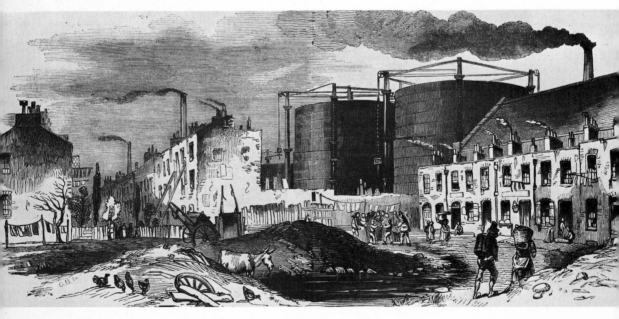

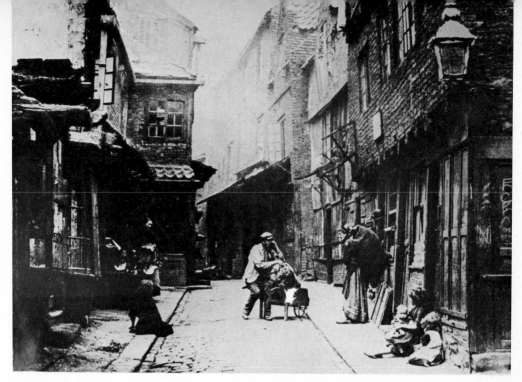

Photograph of Newcastle slums about 1880, showing the dilapidation of the houses and the filth of the streets

Road-sweeper in Chandigarh in India, a new town designed by Le Corbusier to prevent the type of conditions which have made India so susceptible to destructive epidemics

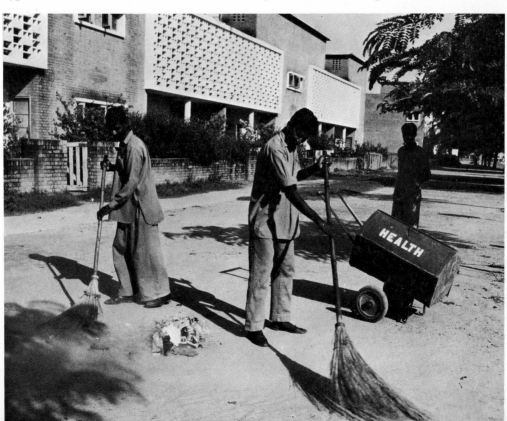

Women in Nigeria crowding to be given a drug to protect their children from meningitis

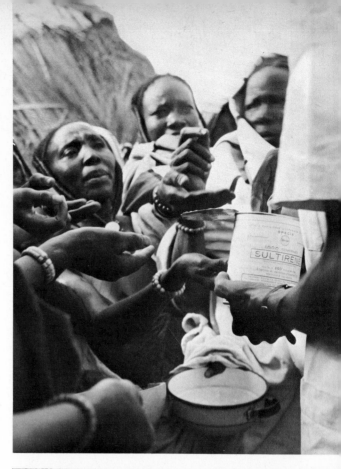

Nigerian child with yaws before and ten days after a single injection of penicillin

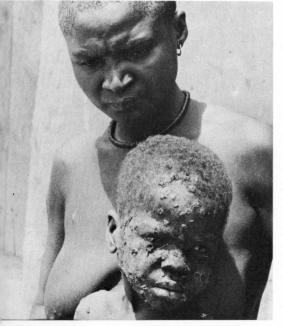

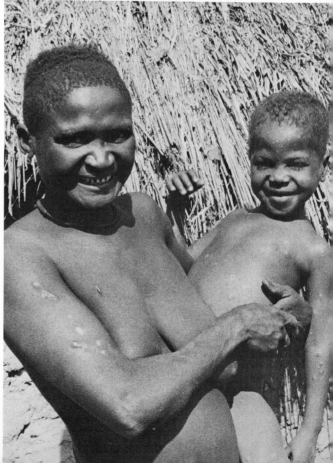

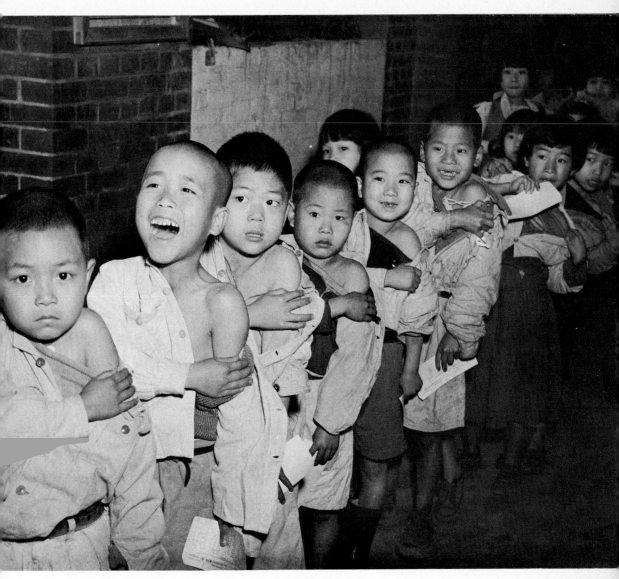

Children in Taiwan queueing up to be inoculated against TB

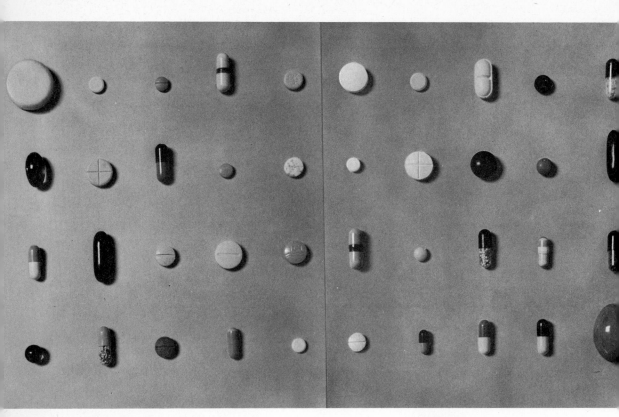

Pills of today: a representative
sample from the 2,000-odd drugs
available on prescription in 1965

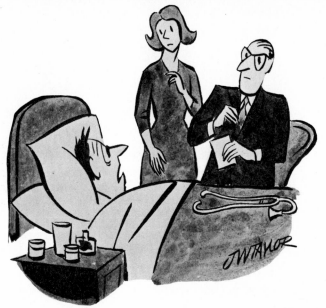

'Drugs, side-effects, more drugs,
more side-effects – couldn't I go
back to the original cold?'

medieval times. Occasionally, an individual doctor made his mark; the most celebrated example being John Snow. In one of the worst outbreaks of cholera that had ever occurred in London, in 1854, some 500 deaths had been reported in ten days from one small area of Soho; and Snow, investigating this geographical oddity, found that nearly all the deaths had taken place within a short distance of a well in Broad Street, off Golden Square. In nearby streets, using a different source, there had been few deaths – and some of them were of children who had been to schools using the Broad Street water. None of the workers in the Broad Street brewery, on the other hand, had died – and Snow found that the brewery had its own well; in any case, the men were given a liquor allowance, and their employer did not think they drank water. The accumulating evidence convinced Snow that the disease must be water-borne; he informed the parish authorities; and 'in consequence of what I said, the handle of the pump was removed on the following day'.

The story of the removal of the Broad Street pump handle is one of the classics in the annals of medical detection; yet the real surprise is not that Snow should have elucidated the truth, by patient investigation, but that it had not been discovered long before. Yet Snow's view was not generally accepted. No medical journal would publish his findings, which he had to bring out at his own expense; it was to be many years before disorders like cholera and typhoid could be brought under control. And in the meantime, though their incidence was much heavier among the poor, they were to carry off many distinguished citizens, including Prince Albert, Queen Victoria's consort, who succumbed to typhoid when he was only forty-two.

With greater economic prosperity, and with the spread of democracy, the reforms which had been urged by men like Frank and Chadwick began to come in piecemeal; and many of the epidemic diseases declined mainly as a result of improved housing and sanitation, long before treatment by any effective drug was available. As Shryock noted, the London County Council was able proudly to boast a nil return for typhus in the annual statistics three years before the transmission route of the disease, through lice, was discovered. In other disorders immunisation could claim much of the credit; particularly in smallpox, where the rate fell sharply wherever vaccination was effectively utilised, and in diphtheria. Here, too, State sanctions had to be invoked. Gradually it came to be accepted that in health matters, the State not only could but should intervene – and not only the State. One of the earliest assumptions of the League of Nations when it was set up after the First World War was that it should concern itself with the prevention and control of disease: and one of the United Nations first actions when it set up a new agency, the World Health Organisation, was by a majority to vote to give it powers (to make quarantine regulations, for example), whereas earlier international bodies had only been advisory.

A few advances in public health were owed to individuals thrusting bureaucratic opposition aside. The development of nursing into a profession owed much to Florence Nightingale; and though she had an influential friend in Sidney Herbert at the War Office, without whose support she would have been powerless to institute her reforms, it was her own vision and drive that carried them through; and without them the hospital system could not have developed, as it was to do, to cater for the sick of every income group on terms of near parity.

The idea of national health services, like the idea of a national education service, was strenuously resisted in some quarters; but it happened that on the issue, conservatism was split. Some conservatives, like Bismarck, believed in compulsory health insurance as a way of killing-socialism-by-kindness; and that was the argument which found general favour in Europe. In Britain after the Second World War it was a Socialist Government that brought in the National Health Service, based on compulsory health insurance for all citizens; but the Conservative Government that followed took care not to disturb the edifice, and even began to claim credit for its smooth running. The medical profession also accepted it, though not without reservations; critics of the NHS, who were becoming more vocal by the 1960s, were less concerned to condemn the principle of a national health service than to point out that such a service might not be necessary in an affluent society, and that it was bureaucratically muscle-bound. In the US, on the other hand, the American Medical Association consistently and often rancorously objected to the whole principle.

Because it is so intimately linked with public health and consequently with politics, preventive medicine has always been the poor relation. In his *History of U.S. Medicine*, Sigerist remarked on the contrast there has so often been between what is known about disease and what is actually done about it: the historian of posterity, he thought, would be astonished, making an analysis of medicine in the first part of the twentieth century, at the contrast between the remarkable advances in curative medicine and the failure to implement them. The student of medical history:

finds that medicine pointed with pride to the number of communicable diseases which were under its control: the bubonic plague, cholera, smallpox, hydrophobia; but he is aware that in all countries thousands of people were still dying every year of preventable diseases, that thousands of children were crippled by rickets, though this disorder could be guarded against, that millions of people suffered from tuberculosis, though there was an accurate knowledge of this disease, that many thousands of women died annually of septic abortion because the law would not permit them to go to a doctor. He learns during his researches that when money was short, the governments curtailed their public health budget. Could people really have been so short-sighted? They spent millions every year for the cure of diseases. Did they not realise that it would less expensive to prevent them?

The only time when preventive medicine really flourished was during wars, when the need to prevent people from falling sick, as distinct from curing them when they did, was urgent. It took conscription in the First World War to reveal the depressingly low physical standards of conscripts in many countries; and this was to lead to greater attention later being paid to preventive measures at school age, from physical check-ups to better school meals. Both wars also helped to break down the prejudice against prophylactic measures in connection with venereal disease; and the second even to lead to the extensive employment of psychiatrists to try to find, and prevent, the spread of disabling mental and emotional stresses. But such measures tended to fall into abeyance, or at least to taper off, in peacetime.

Psychiatry

The branch of medicine which took longest to arouse itself from the torpor of centuries was psychiatry: and again, the initial impulse can be traced back to Mesmer.

Elliotson had failed in his attempt to convert his colleagues to a belief in mesmerism chiefly because he had not fully understood the phenomenon; and Esdaile concentrated on its anaesthetic effects. But meanwhile another Scot, James Braid, was examining the phenomenon in his practice; from his investigation he came to the conclusion that there was a state of mind which he called 'nervous sleep'; and he coined the term hypnotise to describe how it was induced. This type of hypnotism, he insisted, should not be confused with mesmerism. It was not the product of an occult force, animal magnetism: it was subjective, arising from a relationship between hypnotiser and patient – a relationship which could be exploited for purposes of medical treatment.

Braid, too, was unable to convince his colleagues. Like the originators of all new views, he complained, he had suffered much for his contentions, 'for the sceptics, from not perceiving the difference between my method and that of the mesmerists, were equally hostile to hypnotism as they had been to mesmerism; and the mesmerists, thinking their craft was in danger – that their mystical idol was threatened – to be shorn of some of its glory by the advance of a new rival – buckled on their armour, and soon proved that the *odium mesmericum* was as inveterate as the *odium theologicum*'. So the opportunity to explore the new region of the mind which Braid had opened up by hypnotism was not taken.

But by this time, the hypnotic trance state was beginning to arouse interest in France. Jean Charcot's investigations at the Salpêtrière represented a reversion to mesmerism, through which he demonstrated that it could result in artificially induced hysteria, in which patients mimicked disorders they did not have; and this explained much that had previously been mystifying, including manifestations which had earlier been attributed to witchcraft. The symptoms of hysteria could now be observed, and accounted for rationally, even if the mechanism by which the disorders were transmitted remained uncertain. But Charcot missed the therapeutic possibilities of hypnotism; so although he gave the trance state respectability, by proving to the satisfaction of his professional colleagues that it existed, he also enabled them to put it out of their minds. Hysterics, it was believed, were not *really* ill; so their symptoms were regarded as of no more than curiosity value.

A. A. Liébeault, however, a French country doctor, began to use hypnotism in treatment when, having experimented with it out of curiosity, he found it was ideally suited to his practice. Bramwell, the historian of hypnotism, went to visit him in 1889, and found the technique Liébeault was using very different from that which had been a feature of the hectic sessions at the Salpêtrière. Liébeault simply put his patients into what appeared to be a gentle sleep, and made therapeutic suggestions to them – that their symptoms would disappear, or that they would sleep better, or digest their food more easily; off they then went, often claiming to be cured already. Liébeault, it seemed, had found no difficulty in winning acceptance for the method, because he had traded on peasant parsimony. 'If you wish me to treat you with drugs, I will do so, but you will have to pay me as formerly. On the other hand, if you will allow me to hypnotise you, I will do it for nothing.' And having no great ambition, *le bon père Liébeault* kept his word.

This meant that he worked virtually unnoticed for twenty years until, when he moved to Nancy, one of his cures attracted the attention of Hippolyte Bernheim, who had previously treated the patient without success. Bernheim, a professor with an already established reputation in the profession, at first suspected trickery; but when his investigations convinced him that Liébeault's method was genuine, he became a convert, using it countless times himself and collecting evidence from other sources for his *De la Suggestion*. It was published in 1886, and helped finally to establish the method – though orthodoxy continued to view it with suspicion.

Bernheim was not greatly given to theorising, but he did produce one idea that has been nagging away at the conscience of the community ever since. His work on hypnosis, he argued, had disabused him of the notion that the will was a free agent in connection either with neurosis, or with crime; because frequently the will was the helpless slave of the imagination – as it is in hypnotised subjects. 'We are all potentially or actually hallucinating people during most of our lifetimes . . . suggestion, no matter where it comes from, imposes itself on our minds and plays a part in almost all crimes.'

To Bernheim, therefore, can be traced one of the origins of the legal concept now accepted in many a criminal code, of 'diminished responsibility'; the acceptance that psychopaths, men who are morally rather than mentally disordered, should nevertheless be regarded as patients and not as criminals. From this, as Barbara Wootton argued in her *Social Science and Social Pathology*, it is a short step to the corollary, that *all* crime must be treated as disease, and all criminals as patients; because there is not, and cannot be, any way of differentiating between the psychopath and the 'true' criminal. The Scandinavian countries have moved some way towards acceptance of this thesis; a movement which, if it continues, will be revolutionary in its implications for medicine.

The direct influence of Liébeault and Bernheim was relatively small; but their work interested Emile Coué, a young student of chemistry who went to Nancy to watch it in the 1880s, and who was eventually to acquire a far wider fame than they had done. Coué became convinced that the actual therapeutic effort was made not by the hypnotist but by the subject: what was effective, therefore, was really auto-suggestion; and if people knew how to hypnotise themselves, there would be no necessity for the hypnotist. The method he evolved required the recitation of a formula, 'every day, in every way, I get better and better'; and for a time in the 1920s it caught on as a world-wide craze, like contract bridge.

The craze was soon forgotten, and with it Coué; but he had made one contribution – or elaboration on Bernheim's work – the importance of which it is difficult to over-estimate. It is the imagination that is dominant, he insisted, and not the will. 'I get better' was to be regarded not as an order to the mind (which is apt to ignore orders of that kind) but a pronouncement by and for the imagination, because a person who imagines himself better, *is* better. In this, Coué came close to explaining the success of magico-religious practices in medicine. They were not just hopelessly misguided superstition and quackery; they had often been the most effective, and sometimes the only, weapon in medicine's hands; and there was still a place for them in medicine at every level, but particularly in general practice.

Another researcher who received his original inspiration from hypnotism – and was destined to be far more influential than Coué – was Sigmund Freud. A neurologist, Freud became interested in hypnotism when his friend Josef Breuer used it to treat a case of hysteria, 'Anna O', by putting Anna into a trance and encouraging her to talk. She did, freely; and in the process not merely recalled past traumatic events, but felt the emotions which had been connected with them – thereby achieving what Breuer called catharsis, and temporarily losing her hysterical symptoms.

Intrigued, Freud examined the phenomena of hypnotism under Charcot, in Paris, and in 1899 he went to watch the practitioners in Nancy: 'I witnessed the moving spectacle', he wrote in his autobiography, 'of old Liébeault working among the poor women and children of the labouring classes; I was a spectator of Bernheim's astonishing experiments upon his hospital patients; and I received the profoundest impression of the possibility that there could be powerful mental processes which nevertheless remained hidden from the consciousness of men.' Thus was forged the final link in the chain, Mesmer–Charcot–Liébeault–Bernheim–Freud: 'the new psychology', as Zilboorg noted, 'had as little in common with hypnotism as Mesmer with animal magnetism. Yet the chain was not fortuitous; it was made up of therapeutic links.'

Freud began his investigations into the unconscious by using Breuer's methods; but he had to abandon them because, on his own admission, he was not a good hypnotiser. For his later career it was as well that he did – hypnosis would only have confused the issues that he was destined to disentangle; but without its initial assistance he could not have made the discoveries which set him on his path. It was not necessary, he found, to hypnotise patients in order to persuade them to release the flow of recollection. Relaxed on a couch, they could be induced to do so with the same results as Breuer had obtained: recall of repressed thoughts, catharsis and disappearance of symptoms. Sometimes symptoms would return, a signal that not all the material that had been dammed up in the unconscious mind had been released; but if this release could be achieved, the patient would be restored to health. Freud's thesis, in short, was that Eve had been right to eat the apple from the tree of knowledge; and though Carl Jung, for one, disagreed that the serpent (or phallus) played as significant a part in the affair as Freud believed, he agreed about the need for self-knowledge – and not simply on the conscious level; as Freud emphasised, there is 'knowing' and 'knowing'; unless the conscious knowledge is reinforced by related feeling it may be useless.

The importance of Freud's discovery is now generally conceded even by those psychiatrists who disagree with his interpretation of it, and the uses he put it to. 'It was the first time', Zilboorg, again, claimed, 'in the history of psychopathology that the cause of illness, the symptoms generated by the cause, and the therapeutic agent revealing and removing the cause were combined in one succession of factors. It is doubtful whether the full meaning of this historical fact has as yet been properly appreciated. It was this combination that made clinical psychopathology a true medical discipline for the first time in the history of medicine's struggle for the incorporation of neuroses and psychoses into its field of scientific investigation and treatment.'

As treatment, however, Freudian analysis proved disappointing. It took too long; it cost too much; its results were uncertain. For a while orthodox

Freudians tried to hold to the strict analytic procedure, but breakaway movements began; Jung, Alfred Adler and other disciples went their own way, some forming cults of their own. The divisions between the analytic groups, however, no longer appear as deep as they did, because all except a few diehards have accepted the need to modify and adapt analysis for psychotherapy – a term hard to define, because it has been applied to many different procedures; but generally used to describe techniques derived from analysis. The therapist seeks to persuade his patients to talk out their neurosis, and thereby to acquire the insights that will enable them to handle it.

The other theory to influence twentieth-century psychiatry was behaviourist, stemming from Descartes and popularised by the researches of I. P. Pavlov in Russia. Pavlov found that he was able to produce experimental neurosis in dogs by conditioning them to certain expectations – as it might be, food when a bell was rung – and then confusing them by producing different responses – an electric shock instead of the food. From this, it was a short step to wondering whether the cause of neuroses in humans might be a failure to adapt in similar disturbing situations: and the American J. B. Watson, proceeded to verify the theory experimentally. He conditioned a boy who had previously been fond of animals into a phobia about white rats, by loudly banging an iron bar with a hammer just behind the boy whenever he reached out to touch them. It was possible, Watson and later researchers found, both to condition and de-condition people in this way; and this aroused hopes that neuroses and phobias would eventually be eliminated by suitable de-conditioning techniques.

The behaviourist school attracted a vigorous protagonist in H. J. Eysenck of London University, who argued that whereas there was no convincing experimental evidence for the effectiveness of either Freudian or eclectic psychotherapy, conditioning could be shown to work, if it were given a reasonable trial; and experiments were conducted on quite an extensive scale – for example, by giving alcoholics a drug which would make them violently sick whenever they took a drink; or showing male homosexuals pictures of attractive men while subjecting them to unpleasant experiences – electric shocks or nausea. But although successes were claimed, the behaviourist method turned out to have many limitations.

Meanwhile, though, orthodox psychiatry was making advances which owed little to Pavlov or Freud.

The nineteenth century had been a melancholy period for the mentally disordered. The ideas that Tuke, Rush and Pinel had put forward were disregarded. One name stands out: Dorothea Dix, who was so shocked by what she saw when she visited a mental institution in Massachusetts that she devoted the rest of her life to agitating for better conditions for the insane. In her appeal to the legislature of Massachusetts, written in 1843, she expressed her regret that she would have 'to reveal many things revolting to the taste, and from which my woman's nature shrinks with peculiar sensitiveness' but she must tell what she had seen: insane people 'in *cages, closets, cellars, stalls, pens! Chained, naked, beaten with rods and lashed into obedience!*' But her efforts had one unfortunate result. She was able to arouse public conscience, to make even legislators share her horror that the insane should be locked away with inmates of workhouses and prisons. But this led to an even worse fate for the insane: they were locked away in remote institutions behind high walls.

These asylums at first seemed an improvement, but they were in effect prisons, with the additional horror that once inside them the patient could not look forward, as the convict could, to a terminal date on which he would be released. Inside, even those men and women whose insanity would ordinarily have been of short duration might find themselves permanently incarcerated – with the straitjacket and the padded cell if in desperation they lost control of themselves – as Clifford Beers so vividly described in his autobiography, *A Mind that Found Itself*, published in 1908.

Beers' book helped to arouse American public opinion once more to the condition of the insane; and this led to the foundation in the US of the National Committee for Mental Hygiene the following year. The improvement in mental hospitals, though, was not lasting, because the numbers of institutionalised mentally ill began to increase. This was partly because the line where mental disorder could be publicly tolerated was re-drawn; and thousands of men and women who would previously have been allowed to remain with their families were sent to institutions. But it was also because the institutions themselves, it was later realised, created the conditions in which insanity flourished.

Occasionally individual mental hospitals reverted to what came to be known as the 'Open Door' system, allowing patients to feel at liberty; but it was only when electric shock treatment came into use, later to be supplemented by the introduction of 'tranquillisers', that it became general. At last psychiatrists and mental nurses felt they had a real prospect of curing patients who previously had been deemed incurable. At last, the psychiatrist could treat his patients, as distinct from simply keeping them under control; this gave him a real interest in them: they responded; and the resultant interplay of hope and enthusiasm was responsible for the astonishing transformation that came over many mental hospitals after the Second World War.

By the 1960s, though, the gratifying rate of cures in mental hospitals, measured by the percentage of patients considered well enough to be released, was being overhauled by the readmission rate, as ex-patients found the strains and traumas of the outside world too much for them. The old hopelessness, and the old stigma, of mental illness had been broken down; but much more remained to be done. The numbers of psychiatrists and psychiatric auxiliaries remained far too small in relation to the need; and many potentially valuable aids – hypnotherapy, being an obvious example – were hard to introduce because there were insufficient research funds and not enough practitioners. It was becoming clear, too, that an accusation that had been levelled at the tranquillising drugs – that their real benefit was to arouse the psychiatrists rather than to cure the patients – was not far off the mark; tests with controls revealed that a placebo was often as effective. And a prolonged controlled study in Canada of the effects of the brain operation of leucotomy revealed in 1964 that patients who had it had done no better than those who had not.

'There is a wide divergence of diagnosis,' the authors of *Three Hundred Years of Psychiatry*, Richard Hunter and Ida MacAlpine, admitted, 'a steady flow of new terms and an ever-changing nomenclature, as well as a surfeit of hypotheses which tend to be presented as fact. Furthermore, etiology remains speculative, pathogenesis largely obscure, classification predominantly symptomatic and hence arbitrary and possibly ephemeral; physical treatments are empirical and subject to fashion, and psychotherapies still only in their infancy and doctrinaire.' The advances in the treatment of the mentally ill, encouraging though they have been, have represented only a tentative beginning.

Stress and Disease

The advances and the setbacks in the campaign for mental health were experienced in a self-contained, isolated sector of the health campaign. Medical

students usually received nothing that could seriously be described as psychiatric teaching, and what little they learnt was calculated to impress on
them that disorders of the mind were separate from, and largely unrelated
to, disorders of the body. They might occasionally hear a lecturer emphasise
the importance of treating the whole man, mind and body; but in actual
clinical instruction the mind by the 1920s was all but excluded, except in
hysterical and what were called functional – not stemming from any organic
cause – disorders. And hysterical and functional disorders were not regarded
as within the doctor's province: they were thought to show that the patient,
whether aware of it or not, was a malingerer: not really ill.

The interest, then, lay in the treatment of physical disorders with chemical
means. The concept of the importance of the terrain was forgotten. Patients
and doctors thought of diseases as entities spread by disease agents, for which
a cure would eventually be found: a new magic bullet or, better still, a new
wonder drug with a wide range of anti-bacterial action. So far was the significance of the terrain, and in particular of the patient's emotional problems,
neglected that a few doctors who continued to insist upon them had come to
be regarded as cranks.

Freud's discoveries, however, when they began to attract attention after
the First World War, helped to provide an explanation why emotional conditions could cause or precipitate illness. It was not that the patient wanted
to be ill, consciously; but that he was the victim of unconscious processes
militating against health.

In retrospect, it seems barely credible that the influence of mind on body
should have been so far forgotten. Hippocrates had been aware of it; so
were the great Arab doctors of the Moslem empire; so was Paracelsus. More
surprisingly, Harvey himself had emphasised it:

I was acquainted with another strong man, who having received an injury and
affront from one more powerful than himself, and upon whom he could not have
his revenge, was so overcome with hatred and spite and passion, which he yet
communicated to no one, that at last he fell into a strange distemper, suffering from
extreme oppression and pain of the heart and breast and in the course of a few
years died. His friends thought him poisoned by some maleficent influence, or
possessed with an evil spirit . . . In the dead body I found the heart and aorta so
much gorged and distended with blood, that the cavities of the ventricles equalled
those of a bullock's heart in size. Such is the force of the blood pent up, and such

are the effects of its impulse . . . We also observe the signal influence of the affec-
tions of the mind when a timid person is arrested, a deadly pallor overspreads the
surface, the limbs stiffen, the ears sing, the eyes are dazzled or blinded, and, as it
were, convulsed. But here I come upon a field where I might roam freely and give
myself up to speculation. And, indeed, such a flood of light and truth breaks in
upon me here; occasion offers of explaining so many problems, of resolving so
many doubts, of discovering the causes of so many slighter and more serious diseases, and of suggesting remedies for their cure, that the subject seems almost to
demand a separate treatise . . .

. . . And what indeed is more deserving of attention than the fact that in almost
every affection, appetite, hope or fear, our body suffers, the countenance changes,
and the blood appears to course hither and thither. In anger the eyes are fiery and
pupils contracted; in modesty the cheeks are suffused with blushes; in fear, and
under a sense of infamy and of shame, the face is pale, but the ears burn as if for the
evil they heard or were to hear; in lust how quickly is the member distended with
blood and erected!

Intimations of awareness of the mind–body relationship continued – particularly in the case of TB. The American psychiatrist, Hack Tuke published
a series of articles, *Illustrations of the Influence of the Mind upon the Body in
Health and Disease*, revealing its extent and range, in the 1870s. Yet, though
some individuals continued to have reservations, by the end of the century it
was growing rare to encounter references to the possibility of the mind having any but a marginal effect on the body.

The first man to revive the old way of thinking was Georg Groddeck. He
had been an orthodox physician – for a time he was in charge of a military
hospital at Baden Baden; but observation suggested to him that disease is not,
as he had been taught to assume, the result of a single cause, but of many
causes, among them the patient's way of, and attitude to, life; and this led
him to admire Freud's work, and realise its significance, when he came across
it. Man, he wrote, 'creates his own illnesses for definite purposes, using the
outer world merely as an instrument'. The doctor, therefore, must ask himself not, 'What caused this illness?' but 'What are the symptoms trying to tell
me?' No drug, however potent, would provide a lasting cure: only the
establishment of a therapeutic *rapport* between patient and doctor, which
Groddeck considered more important than anything else in handling disease.
But he was one of those larger-than-life characters who make more impact

on a small circle of acquaintances and patients than on posterity; his writings did not attract a large public.

More influential as a publicist was Flanders Dunbar, whose *Mind and Body: Psychosomatic Medicine*, appeared in 1947. For many of its readers it must have been the earliest intimation of what 'psychosomatic' meant – or even of its existence: and she provided an impressive range of case histories to show how emotional disturbance, often stemming from childhood, could be the root cause of stomach ulcers, asthma, heart disease, allergies, and even accidents. But the book was too readably written to impress the profession: and it was some time before the term 'psychosomatic' was accepted in medical journals without the protective quotation marks around it, as if it was not yet to be trusted.

For the profession, the decisive step towards making psychosomatic medicine acceptable – though the process was to last years – had been taken in the experiment on 'Tom' a New York hospital janitor who, following a childhood accident, had to be fed through a pipe directly into his stomach – giving the same opportunity that had presented itself to William Beaumont to make experiments on the digestive process. Beaumont had noticed that it could be influenced by the trapper's emotional state; on March 12, 1830, his trapper had had a breakfast of fat pork, bread and potatoes, and at lunchtime Beaumont observed that the digested meal was 'considerably tinged with yellow bile; a circumstance which I had but once before observed in my experiments on him. And this I supposed to have been the effect of violent anger.' But it was over a century before two of the doctors in the hospital in which 'Tom' worked took up where Beaumont had left off, testing 'Tom's' stomach reactions to such emotions as annoyance and worry. They found that alarm over the prospect of the loss of his job was reflected in the state of his stomach's lining; it became fragile, so that slight friction caused it to bleed. There could hardly have been a more convincing example of the importance of the terrain in illness, for in ordinary circumstances 'Tom' had a healthy digestion; when under emotional stress he became, in effect, ulcer prone.

At this time the psychosomaticists, as they sometimes apologetically called themselves, had mostly been concentrating on establishing links between disorders and emotional predisposition along Freudian lines; Flanders Dunbar thought of asthma as representing the repressed cry of a child, craving love. But the work on 'Tom' suggested other possibilities, and they were followed up by Hans Selye in Montreal, with experiments on rats. Selye's theory, described in *The Stress of Life*, went back to the homeostatic process outlined by Claude Bernard. The life force, Selye argued, coped with threats to the constitution by mobilising the body's defences, the glands playing an all-important part. The symptoms of our illness, as Sydenham had realised, are often merely the signs that the mobilisation has been effected, and that the troops have gone into action. But if the life force is distracted, it may not be able to function satisfactorily; and in his best-known experiment, Selye showed that animals given a dose of hormones that ordinarily they could have thrown off without difficulty were killed by it if, at the same time, they were subjected to the equivalent of frustration. If they were tied down to a board

large patches of their heart muscle underwent acute disintegration, and all the animals died within a few hours. Animals not pretreated with these hormones withstand the same frustrating experience without difficulty ... All these observations have been confirmed in the primate (rhesus monkey); this suggests that man is likely to respond similarly under comparable conditions. Attention is called to the fact that in its microscopic features, the cardiac damage produced under these conditions in experimental animals is quite similar to that seen in men who die from an acute cardiac accident as a result of exposure to stress.

The stress theory of disease redressed the balance that had been upset by the germ theory. It showed that the humoralists had been right, and that Pettenkofer had not been a lucky exception: any really healthy man, free from stress, might have drunk off that cholera potion and lived. Not that stress as such was harmful, as Selye was careful to insist; on the contrary, it was an essential ingredient of life. But unduly prolonged or unnecessary stress, and in particular that caused by repressed emotional trauma, could be the real cause of disease and death, even when a specific virus or poison was found; because without the stress, they would have been powerless to harm.

This could apply even in the case of epidemics. From his experience of tropical medicine in India, A. T. W. Simeons cited Asiatic cholera as an example, in his *Man's Presumptuous Brain*:

Working in the midst of an epidemic outbreak of cholera one cannot help noticing the strange fact that the healthy adolescent, the busy mother and the wage-earning father are more often stricken than the very young children and the old and decrepit. Cholera is caused by swallowing a microbe called a vibrio and it is known that the cholera vibrio is highly sensitive to acids. The acid that is always present in the normal human stomach is sufficiently strong to kill the cholera vibrio almost instantly. How then does the vibrio overcome this acid barrier which separates it from the small intestines where, in the alkaline contents, it can thrive and start its murderous activity?

The answer seems to be that it cannot. Only if the normal flow of acid in the stomach is shut off is the vibrio able to reach its destination. Now the one thing that stops the flow of acid in the stomach is fear and panic. So it may come about that those most terrified of death are just the ones the cholera kills, while those too young to understand the danger and those to whom life seems hardly worth living and who fatalistically tend the sick and dying around them, may survive unscathed, because the secretion of their gastric juice is not emotionally inhibited. Fear might thus play an important role in the selection of victims, and in this sense it would not be incorrect to say that even in cholera psychosomatic mechanisms can be of importance. Similar factors may be involved in the sudden onset of some cases of bacillary dysentery or in typhoid fever – but not in plague, where the bacillus is injected straight into the blood by the bite of a rat flea.

The stress theory of disease promised a medical revolution even more far-reaching in its effects than its microbiological predecessor. For if the import-ance of the terrain, and particularly the patient's emotional condition, were to be conceded, changes would be required not merely in the medical cur-riculum – still basically mechanistic and physical in orientation – but even more in the selection of doctors, who would require a very different outlook to understand, diagnose and treat stress disorders. The trend away from gen-eral practice to specialisation would also have to be reversed; for only by a return to the family doctor, old style, who knew his patients and their cir-cumstances (and not just their symptoms), could the appropriate preventive measures be undertaken.

II

THE 1960s

WE usually think of rationalism as the characteristically progressive element, fighting against superstition and irrationalism where the latter have become the habitual bulwark of entrenched irrational privilege . . . But there have existed perhaps quite other situations, in which mysticism has played the part of a progressive social force. When a certain body of rationalist thought has become irrevocably tied to a rigid and outdated system of society, and has become associated with the social controls and sanctions which it imposes, then mysticism may become revolutionary.

The writer – Joseph Needham – was recalling medical upheavals in ancient China and in Europe; with particular reference to van Helmont, one of the founders of biochemistry, and yet 'deeply anti-rational'. But the theory applies with equal force to the present day. 'Scientific' medicine, of the narrow, rationalist kind, is almost exhausted. It is continually claiming victory on this or that sector of the health front; but over the front as a whole there is no longer advance.

One reason can be found in the adoption, a century ago, of too rigidly materialist a conception of disease. Since it has been found that placebo effect was a measurable therapeutic aid, the foundations of what has passed for rational medicine have begun to crumble. True, orthodoxy never denied the potential of suggestion, but they failed to grasp its significance, and made no attempt to exploit it.

The second mistake has been to underestimate the importance of biology, as compared with pathology and chemistry. 'If the introduction of the cowpox should extirpate the smallpox', Malthus wrote in his *Essay on Population*, 'we shall find increased mortality of some other diseases.' Events have proved his point. Chemotherapy has banished or brought under control many diseases; but there are no signs of a reduction of disease in general. To some extent, admittedly, overcrowded surgeries and hospital wards can be accounted for by the fact there are more old people to get ill; to some extent, by greater affluence – though in some ways it may help people to be healthier, it also encourages them to visit a doctor with less concern about the expense. But even making such allowances, the disease rate is still disturbingly high – particularly for mental illness.

The most serious error, though, into which orthodox medicine has fallen is too narrowly to restrict the confines of science. The tendency has been to insist that whatever is not seen or not understood does not exist. The obvious example is hypnotism, derided and rejected by the profession for more than a century after it was first discovered, and to this day only tolerated – rarely explored, and not taught at medical schools.

Mesmerism was rejected because it smacked of mysticism – of the occult; and even today, most doctors who accept it, at least in its refined form of hypnotism, still reject the idea of animal magnetism, and regard such practitioners as Paracelsus, Greatraks and Elisha Perkins as either deluded or frauds. Yet in 1963 *Nature* published the findings of two researchers in Utah State University, Dr A. A. Boe and Dr D. K. Salunkhe, who had experimented by growing tomatoes between two strong magnetic poles, with control plants for purposes of comparison; and the magnetised plants grew much faster than the controls. As for Mesmer's occultism, in 1964 Dr Marcel Poumailloux told the British Medical Association's conference that a prolonged study of 'coronaries' in France had shown that they seemed to increase after sunstorms – connected, apparently, with the increase in cosmic rays striking the earth. Research in the US, too, has suggested that the onset of mental disorder is also often related to extra-terrestrial activity (the term 'lunatic' may turn out not to be so misleading, after all) and the United States Department of Health, Education and Welfare has pronounced, 'there is enough evidence for expert research into health indications in a person's palm' – following an earlier assertion in the *Lancet* that the palms have 'great diagnostic value'.

These are not symptoms of a regression into superstition: they are mysticism in its revolutionary role, seeking not so much to overturn established science as to enlarge its boundaries. The old materialism has in any case been exploded with the discovery of nuclear energy: apart from the fact that it has posed problems which cannot be solved by old-style physics, it has also destroyed the distinction between matter and energy, and revealed how little is yet known about energy in, among other things, its therapeutic capacity.

At the same time, the experiments of Rhine, Soal and others, by helping to shift extra-sensory perception from an anecdotal on to an experimental basis, have made it impossible any longer to reject the idea of mind-transmitted healing. If it is conceded (as it has been by many scientists who have studied the subject with no sceptical holds barred) that telepathic communication can be established, and if it is also accepted, as it must be, that suggestion is an extremely powerful therapeutic force, then it has to be realised that health (or sickness) may be transmitted from one person to another, at a distance, by suggestion telepathically delivered. As yet this can only be regarded as a hypothesis; but it fits the observed facts, and makes sense of much that used to be inexplicable except in terms of superstition.

There is no question of repudiating the work of Pasteur, Koch and their successors. Microbes and viruses are often a cause, and sometimes *the* cause, of disease. But they are rarely the only cause; and for the purpose of preventing disease, and even to some extent of treating it, all the other possible causal agents – evolution and constitution, heredity and environment, stresses external and internal – need to be taken into consideration; and, consequently, anything that exerts a therapeutic force – even if to admit it appears 'unscientific' in the recently held definition of that term – has to be considered.

It is not enough, then, to say, 'all right: perhaps there is such a thing as telepathy: perhaps there is such a thing as a healing force which can be transmitted, even to a distance: but until it is found let us continue with our operations and our drugs.' If the force is there, it needs to be investigated. It has not, and is not now, being investigated by the profession; except peripherally. Even placebo effect, though it has been so amply demonstrated, is still generally regarded as an unfortunate impediment, a nuisance rather than a valuable therapeutic ally; and 'healing' has become almost a term of reproach, used about the work of unorthodox practitioners. These and other practices – hypnosis, acupuncture, manipulation, divination and many more – require to be more systematically and sympathetically investigated and understood, if we are to begin to comprehend the mystery of disease.

BIBLIOGRAPHY

Secondary sources referred to or quoted from in the text. The date given is of the edition that I have consulted.

Browne, Edward G., *Arabian Medicine* (Cambridge, 1921)

Buchanan, Scott, *The Doctrine of Signatures* (London, 1938)

Buck, Albert, *The Growth of Medicine* (Yale, 1917)

Calder, Ritchie, *Medicine and Man* (London, 1958)

Dubos, René, *Louis Pasteur* (London, 1951)

Dunbar, Flanders, *Mind and Body* (New York, 1955)

Eysenck, H. J., *Uses and Abuses of Psychology* (London, 1955)

Garrison, Fielding H., *Introduction to the History of Medicine* (London, 1929)

Ghalioungui, Paul, *Magic and Medical Science in Ancient Egypt* (London, 1963)

Guirdham, A., *A Theory of Disease* (London, 1957)

Guthrie, Douglas, *A History of Medicine* (London, 1958)

Haggard, Howard W., *The Doctor in History* (Yale, 1934)

Hargrave, John, *The Life and Soul of Paracelsus* (London, 1951)

Hecker, J. F. C., *The Epidemics of the Middle Ages* (London, 1859)

Horder, Lord, *Fifty Years of Medicine* (London, 1953)

Hunter, Richard, and MacAlpine, Ida, *Three Hundred Years of Psychiatry* (Oxford, 1963)

Jameson, Eric, *The Natural History of Quackery* (London, 1961)

Koestler, Arthur, *The Sleepwalkers* (London, 1959)

Lasagna, Louis, *The Doctor's Dilemmas* (New York, 1962)

Leff, S. & V., *From Witchcraft to World Health* (London, 1956)

Lockhart Mummery, J. P., *Nothing New under the Sun* (London, 1947)

Munthe, Axel, *The Story of San Michele* (London, 1930)

Olmsted, J. M. D. and E. H., *Claude Bernard* (New York, 1961)

Osler, William, *The Evolution of Modern Medicine* (Oxford, 1921)

Pauwels, Louis, and Bergier, Jacques, *Le Matin des Magiciens* (Paris, 1960)

Risley, Mary, *The House of Healing* (London, 1962)

Rivers, W. H. R., *Medicine, Magic and Religion* (London, 1924)

Robinson, Victor, *The Story of Medicine* (New York, 1931)

Sargant, W., *Battle for the Mind* (London, 1954)

Selye, Hans, *The Stress of Life* (London, 1956)

Sigerist, Henry, *A History of Medicine* (Oxford, 1951)

Simeons, A. T. W., *Man's Presumptuous Brain* (London, 1960)

Singer, Charles, and Underwood, E. Ashworth, *A Short History of Medicine* (Oxford, 1962)

Theories and Philosophies of Medicine, Institute of History of Medicine and Medical Research (Delhi, 1962)

Underwood, E. A. (ed.), *Science, Medicine and History* (Oxford, 1953)

Wesley, John, *Primitive Physick* (Bristol, 1768)

Williams, Harley, *The Healing Touch* (London, 1949)

Withington, E. T., *Medical History from the earliest times* (London, 1894)

Wootton, A. C., *Chronicles of Pharmacy* (London, 1910)

Zilboorg, Gregory, *A History of Medicine* (New York, 1941)

Zinsser, Hans, *Rats, Lice and History* (New York, 1934)

INDEX

Abortion, 171
abracadabra, 79–80
abreaction, 8, 29
Académie des Sciences, 97, 122–4
acupuncture, 13–15, 186
Adler, Alfred, 176
Admiralty, the, 114, 115
Aesculapius, 22
temples of, 22–4, 57, 61
after life, 12, 61
Aknahton, 21
Albert, Prince, death of, 169
Albucasis, 46, 84, 85
alchemists, 45, 76, 78–9
alchemy, 44–5, 78
alcoholics, 176
Alexander of Tralles, 49, 51
Alexandria, 33–5, 41, 67
allergies, 159, 181
allopathy, 33, 34, 101, 124
amputation, 73, 84, 147
amulets, 20, 37, 50, 51, 62, 80, 90
anaesthetics, 87, 150, 153, 154, 159
discovery of, 145, 147–9
anaesthetists, 149
anaphylactic shock, 159
anatomy, study of, 17, 34, 37, 81–3, 87, 98, 128
pathological, 154
anemia, 160
angina pectoris, 164
animals, 1, 3, 58, 142

animals—contd
diseases in, 2–3
healing in, 4
instinct in, 4, 5
dissection of, 81, 82, 83
experiments on, 157, 158, 160, 176, 182
'Anna O', 91, 174
anthrax, 125, 156, 158
antibiotics, 160–2, 163
antisepsis, 151–2
anti-toxins, 160
apothecaries, 69, 70, 75, 93, 134, 135–7, 138
Society of, 136
Arabs, 41–2, 44–6, 47–8
archeus, see life force
Aristotle, 31, 32, 43, 68
armies, epidemics in, 89, 90, 115–16, 158
army surgeons, 85, 127, 150, 158
arthritis, 10, 15, 162, 163
Asclepiades, 27, 32–3, 105
asepsis, 87, 149–50, 152–4
Asoka, Prince, 57–8, 59
Assurbanipal, King, library of, 16
asthma, 159, 181–2
astrology, 16, 68, 70, 96, 97, 100
astronomy, 74
Auenbrugger, Leopold, 126
Aurelius, Marcus, 35, 37
auscultation, 126–7
Avenzoar, 47

Averroes, 47
Avicenna, 42, 43–4, 84, 150
Canon of, 43, 48
mentioned, 46, 54, 70, 72, 73, 82

Babylon, 15–16, 22, 40, 51, 52, 150, 165
bacilli, 63, 156, 158, 183
Bacon, Francis, 97
Bacon, Roger, 71
bacteriology, 151, 164–5
anti-bacterial drugs, 160, 161, 165, 179
see also germs, microbes
Baglivi, Giorgio, 107–8
Banting, Frederick, 160
barber-surgeons, 84, 135
Bassi, Agostino, 155
Beaumont, William, 127–8, 181
Beecher, Henry K., 164
behaviourism, 106, 107, 176
Behring, von, 125, 158, 160
Bentham, Jeremy, 166
Bergmann, Ernst von, 152
Bernard, St, 61
Bernard, Claude, 129–32, 141, 156, 157, 162, 182
Bernheim, Hippolyte, 173–5
Best, Charles, 160
bezoar stone, the, 47
Bible, the, 52, 53, 56, 61
Bichat, Xavier, 129

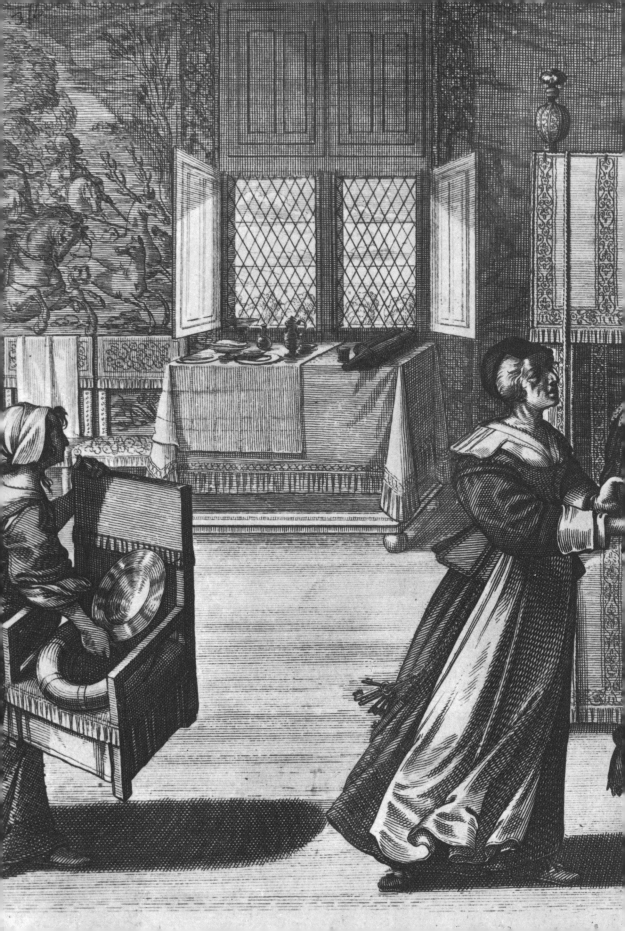